How to Get a Great Night's Sleep

How to Get a Great Night's Sleep

Step-by-step, practical advice for everyone who needs to sleep better.

H. Vafi, M.D. AND Pamela Vafi

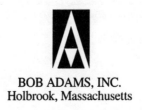

BOB ADAMS, INC.
Holbrook, Massachusetts

Published by Bob Adams, Inc.
260 Center Street, Holbrook, MA 02343

ISBN: 1-55850-442-7

Printed in the United States of America.

J I H G F E D C B A

Library of Congress Cataloging-in-Publication Data
Vafi, H.
How to get a great night's sleep : step-by-step, practical advice for everyone
who needs to sleep better / H. Vafi and Pamela Vafi.
    p.   cm.
Includes index.
ISBN 1-55850-442-7
    1. Sleep—Popular works. 2. Sleep disorders—Popular works. I. Vafi,
Pamela. II. Title.
RA786.V34   1994
616.8'498—dc20   94-32140
CIP

This book is available at quantity discounts for bulk purchases.
For information, call 1-800-872-5627.

To Jeanne,
Al,
Lil,
Roxanne, and
Joe

Contents

Introduction

If you have trouble sleeping at night and rarely awaken feeling refreshed and ready to tackle a new day, you have joined the ranks of over 40 million Americans who report sleeping difficulties. Although the scientific study of sleep is a relative newcomer to the field of medicine, impressive gains have been made since the 1960s. Sleep specialists agree that by improving the quality of your sleep, you will begin to notice positive change in other areas of your life. Daytime functioning improves, life expectancy may increase, and the negative effects of stress and aging diminish.

Specialists emphasize, however, that most insomniacs do have a good deal of stress in their lives and lifestyle changes are typically in order. Improving sleep promotes physical and mental health; however, to improve sleep you must make a committed effort to observe, then challenge the areas in your life that may be responsible for your sleeplessness. Achieving and maintaining optimum health is an active process. You cannot afford to passively ignore your physical and mental health and expect to remain free from disease. Like high blood pressure, high cholesterol, obesity, exercise intolerance, and excess anxiety and anger, prolonged insomnia can lead to deterioration of health and well-being.

Currently over one-half of all illnesses in the United States are lifestyle diseases and are, therefore, potentially preventable. But many look for an easy way out, for something or someone that is going to give them a quick fix or a magic pill. But there is no magic—only a determination to make positive change, and then stick with it.

Achieving wellness, however, does not have to create additional pain; instead, each *small* step you take brings you closer to health and fitness. And that is the key: small steps. Commit to make positive change in your life, but do so slowly and gently. You cannot heal your insomnia the same way you acquired it: with driving energy, a hectic pace, and a negative learning environment that will ultimately undermine your health.

By following the practical techniques and suggestions that comprise the bulk of this text, you can develop the mental power to achieve restful sleep and a more dynamic and healthier approach toward living.

Chapter 1
Understanding How You Sleep

NORMAL SLEEP CYCLES

In this chapter we will explain the normal stages of sleep and the types of insomnia that occur when these sleep cycles are interrupted. By defining what sleep is and how it occurs and clarifying the myths surrounding it, you will have a strong foundation upon which you can successfully apply the techniques that you learn in this book.

Sleep requirements vary dramatically from person to person. Whether you need six or nine hours, the key to refreshing sleep is the cyclic process that begins the moment you drift off to sleep. Understanding the sleep cycles or "stages" of a normal night's sleep the is key to realizing why you may feel better after some nights of interrupted sleep than others, and why sleep cycle deprivation can leave you feeling exhausted.

When the normal sleeper first drifts off to sleep he or she enters Stage 1. This is a shallow state of sleep in which breathing becomes slow and regular and muscles begin to release tension. Brain waves begin to slow down and the person's eyes tend to roll slightly. For the first few minutes of sleep, the brain is producing alpha waves, an electrical wave pattern that indicates a decrease in brain activity.

This decrease in brain activity produces a relaxed, tranquil mental state conducive to deeper relaxation. Stage 1 sleep lasts approximately five minutes and then proceeds to Stage 2. During this stage of sleep a person begins to enter the early phase of deep relaxation. The level of relaxation becomes progressively deeper throughout Stage 2, which typically lasts 45 to 50 minutes. Stage 3 is a brief phase that permits further slowing of brain waves, allowing the individual to proceed to Stage 4 approximately one hour after falling asleep.

Stage 4 brain wave patterns produce delta waves, a very slow pattern associated with the deepest level of sleep. It is during this phase that sleep walking, talking in one's sleep, and night terrors (bad dreams that occur in stage 4 sleep and are characterized by thrashing movement) occur. For the average sleeper this period of deep sleep lasts approximately one hour.

Following Stage 4, brain wave activity begins to increase and progress to an alert active state, producing beta waves, the same brain wave patterns that are present during daytime activities. When experienced during sleep, however, beta wave activity indicates another stage of sleep known as REM, or rapid eye movement. It is during this phase of sleep that pronounced eye movement is noticed and most dreaming occurs. In direct contrast to Stage 4, it is during REM sleep that a person is most easily aroused. If a person is allowed to sleep uninterrupted, however, this period of REM will normally last between 15 and 30 minutes.

If this has been a person's first sleep cycle of the night, he or she will probably repeat this process again. It is likely, however, that the sleeper will enter REM immediately after Stage 3, bypassing Stage 4 for the remainder of the night. The average sleeper completes four or five cycles per night, but the quality of sleep changes the longer the individual remains sleeping. The first cycle of sleep is usually the most sound and has the shortest REM period. During the last half of the night REM increases and becomes much more pronounced.

Although a normal sleep cycle varies from person to person, its average length ranges from a little over an hour to just under two hours. In addition, each person is unique in the number of sleep cycles he or she may need to feel rested the following day. Common to all, however, is the physical response that occurs as each sleeper passes rhythmically from non-REM (Stages 1 through 4) to REM sleep. Notice the specific responses characteristic of non-REM and REM:

Non-REM: Quiet Sleep (Stages 1 through 4)
- No rapid eye movement
- Pulse, respiration, blood pressure normally lowered
- Positional changes occur
- Stages 1 through 4 reflect progressively deeper sleep

REM: Alert/Dreaming Sleep

- Rapid eye movement
- Pulse, respiration, blood pressure fluctuate
- Lack of body movement
- Physiological sexual arousal
- Microscopic muscles in the ear respond as if listening intently

REM Sleep

REM sleep is a unique stage of sleep in which dreaming and sexual arousal occur. It is during this period that males experience erections and females produce vaginal lubrication and swelling. This is a normal process and usually occurs during each REM cycle.

The possibility also exists that dreaming, which occurs during REM, may be a product of the right brain. This offers an explanation for why people rarely spend time calculating numbers or reading while they dream. It is within the left hemisphere of the brain that, while awake, people are able to communicate verbally, balance checkbooks, read a newspaper, or drive a car. The left hemisphere enables people to deal with reality in a concrete manner. The right brain, however, has difficulty reading, working mathematical problems, or understanding language, and may be the seat of the abstract, imagination, and creativity. The right brain often creates the idea behind the fact, allowing the left brain to take that idea and turn it into reality. When a person is awake, the left brain exerts a certain amount of control over the right brain with a blending of skills from both hemispheres. When a person dreams, however, the right brain may assume dominance—which would account for the bizarre content of many people's dreams.

Another phenomena of REM sleep is the occurrence of motor inhibition of voluntary muscles (any muscle over which a person has deliberate and conscious control). Although the body is capable of movement during all other stages of sleep, the dreaming brain protects the body by preventing you from acting out your dreams. In short, your brain prevents your muscles from receiving the messages they need to begin movement. Imagine a dream in which you are swimming or running and the potential for injury if your muscles responded accordingly. And think of the person sleeping next to you. If your muscles were able to move during REM sleep, you would never know what shape you or your partner would be in when you awakened. This is why dreaming during Stage 4 can be dangerous. It is during Stage 4 that sleep walking and talking occur—because there is no REM sleep to inhibit action.

When a dream turns sour in the REM phase of sleep it becomes a nightmare. When you awaken from a nightmare, you can remember the dream and still feel oriented to your surroundings. Nightmares occur during the period of motor inhibition; thus, no acting out of the dream occurs. Typically, nightmares take place during the last half of the night when REM sleep is at its peak. Night terrors, on the other hand, usually occur during the first half of the night when sleep is in its deepest stage. A person who awakens from Stage 4 sleep feels disoriented. She often returns to sleep quickly, and is unable to recall the content of her bad dream. Night terrors produce feelings of intense panic. Since motor inhibition does not occur, thrashing limbs, rapid heartbeat, and confused speech are common during dreaming.

Reticular Activating System
Before the normal sleeper falls asleep, a portion of the brain called the reticular activating system, or RAS, must destimulate. The reticular activating system consists of a group of cells beginning at the top of the spinal cord and terminating in the cerebrum. The cerebrum occupies the major part of the skull cavity. Lying immediately behind the cerebrum, comprising the back portion of the skull cavity, is the cerebellum. It is within the cerebrum, however, that most of an individual's important mental functions occur. The cerebellum is responsible in large part for maintaining equilibrium.

The RAS has two major functions. First, it acts as an alerting mechanism for the brain in much the same way as a knock on the door signals the arrival of a guest. The knock does not tell you who has arrived, merely that someone is seeking entry. Likewise, the RAS doesn't tell a person what the message is, only that some type of stimulation is present. It remains the responsibility of the cortex (the surface area covering the cerebrum that influences thought, feeling, and action) to interpret the alerting stimuli.

The second function of the RAS is to filter the bombardment of incoming stimuli. For example, if you are watching TV, you may not be aware of the furnace kicking on or the sound of passing traffic. Your RAS is not allowing entry of these stimuli to your conscious level of awareness. Filtering unimportant stimuli is a protective mechanism that prevents sensory overload from the constant stimulation of the environment. This filtering process continues even when you sleep. For example, a young mother can sleep through a thunderstorm and yet awaken to the sound of her stirring infant.

The firing rate of the cells within the RAS increases toward alerting stimuli. Conversely, it decreases toward what is unimportant or nonthreatening. Any sudden change in stimulation (such as silence pierced by an infant's cry) alerts a person of potential emergency, and the firing rate increases. If, on the other hand, stimulation becomes constant or is nonthreatening (as with the hum of a fan), the cells of the RAS begin to destimulate. As a result, the brain blocks the particular stimuli from consciousness and ceases to be aware of its sound. If the slowing down process continues, the sleep-promoting centers of the brain eventually activate and sleep follows.

Interestingly, we can train our RAS. We are, however, already somewhat adept at this process. The mere act of growing up and assuming adult responsibility demands that we display less excitability. We learn to focus our attention by gaining mastery over our response to multiple stimuli within our environment. Unlike a small child, an adult can discriminate between what demands attention and what can pass by unnoticed.

WHEN NORMAL SLEEP CYCLES ARE INTERRUPTED

Insomniacs, in general, have a difficult time relaxing and this inability effects their sleep patterns as well. Insomnia, or the prolonged inability to get adequate sleep, can assume a variety of forms, but the effects of sleep deprivation reduce the quality of life for all people alike.

Hyperactive RAS

For most people, sleep is an effortless process. It occurs naturally as their RAS destimulates and the sleep-promoting centers assume dominance. Insomnia, however, is an example of this system gone awry. The insomniac's RAS appears to excite too easily and destimulate too slowly.

A possible cause for this physiological quirk is that insomniacs appear to have excessively stimulated autonomic (involuntary) nervous systems. As a group, insomniacs appear to startle more easily than average people, and their hearts beat faster and harder than those without sleep difficulties. Also, insomniacs report a greater sense of anxiety from stimuli perceived much less stressful by the well-rested. Insomniacs maintain this excessive stimulation during sleep and wakeful states alike. As a result, the overstimulated RAS is unable to filter selectively, which creates a vicious cycle in which the RAS feeds this excessive stimuli back to the autonomic nervous system and cortex (making the person feel more nervous and anxious). In return, the heart beats faster and the mind begins to race, which, in turn, increases the firing rate of the cells within the RAS. And, there you have it, the makings for another sleepless night.

Sound complicated? Imagine, if you will, watching your favorite television program—an enjoyable experience for most people. Now imagine watching that same program with poor reception. The picture and sound are fuzzy and you begin to feel annoyed and frustrated by this unwanted interference. If the interference is great enough, you would probably change channels or turn your television off. This is what occurs when your RAS loses its ability to filter adequately. Unlike your television set, however, you cannot turn it off. As a result, the inability to filter produces an accumulation of interference that results in sensory overload, which, in turn, can produce symptoms of insomnia, anxiety, irritability, or depression.

General Sleep Deprivation
Even after 36 to 46 hours without sleep, most people suffer very few ill effects. After this period, however, most people experience extreme irritability, impulsiveness, and poor problem-solving skills. Judgment becomes impaired and reaction time increases.

If sleep deprivation continues past an average of four or five days, a person will most likely develop symptoms similar to paranoid schizophrenia. She may experience auditory and visual hallucinations, and most likely become paranoid with a marked sense of persecution. Short-term memory becomes impaired and a persistent loss in concentration develops. Unlike schizophrenia, however, the symptoms of even prolonged sleep deprivation subside after a good night's sleep.

Interestingly, even a person deprived of sleep for as many as 9 to 10 days will not need to sleep longer than 16 consecutive hours to awaken feeling refreshed. She will, however, spend a greater than average time in Stage 4 sleep and far less time in the REM phase, since needed biological repair occurs primarily during Stage 4.

Non-REM Deprivation
A deficiency in non-REM sleep is common in some forms of depression. In addition, the pattern of REM cycles appears to alter. In normal sleep stage patterns, the peak REM occurrence is during the latter half of the night. The depressed individual, however, experiences the majority of his REM sleep during the first half of the night. It is also characteristic of the depressed to experience exaggerated rapid eye movement during REM periods.

In addition to altered REM cycles, depressed people frequently experience a reduction in Stages 3 and 4 sleep. As a result, they do not achieve deep sleep and symptoms of insomnia develop. Sleep experts suspect that the heightened REM experience may account for the increased rate of nightmares among the depressed.

REM Deprivation

Many people suffering from insomnia experience a deficiency in REM sleep. When these people do sleep, they do so out of exhaustion and spend inordinate amounts of time in deep Stage 4 sleep. As a result, they experience many of the symptoms associated with REM deficiency.

The symptoms associated with REM deprivation include irritability, hostility, impulsiveness, and short-term memory impairment. The effects vary from person to person. For most, however, aggression and sensitivity to pain increase when REM deficiencies exist. Long-term REM deprivation typically results in a chronic state of moderate to severe functional impairment. Few insomniacs remain unaffected in their ability to maintain a normal and fulfilling lifestyle.

When a normal sleeper is REM deprived for several days, and then allowed to sleep without interruption, he will experience increased dreaming. This is a compensatory mechanism enabling him to catch up on REM sleep. For the chronic insomniac, however, it remains more important to spend what little time he does sleep, sleeping as soundly as possible. Thus, the biological repair that Stage 4 provides is of greater importance than the psychological repair obtained during REM sleep.

Insomnia and high fevers can reduce REM, but so, too, can prescription and over-the-counter sleep aids. Drug-induced REM deficiency also produces next-day crankiness, aggression, pain intolerance, and short-term memory impairment. Thus, a person can suffer symptoms of REM deficiency even after a drug-induced good night's sleep. And should a person stop taking drugs such as sleeping pills, he may find that he begins having nightmares that may last up to a week. In the brain's attempt to catch up on lost REM sleep, excessive and intense dreaming often occur.

MYTHS AND FACTS

There are a variety of common beliefs surrounding sleep that can affect how well-rested you feel when you awaken in the morning. Many myths associated with sleep patterns, sleep habits and insomnia people accept as fact. As you read through the following list, note how many of these myths you, too, accept as fact.

Myth: I should fall asleep immediately after going to bed. If I am still awake after 15 minutes, I have insomnia.

Fact: Sleep normally occurs within 20 to 30 minutes after going to bed. This is a natural and passive slowing down process.

Myth: If I sleep less than seven or eight hours a night, I am not getting sufficient sleep.

Fact: If you sleep five hours nightly and awaken feeling alert and well rested, you have had adequate sleep.

Myth: Occasional alcohol consumption at bedtime will help me sleep better.

Fact: Alcohol induced sleep prevents the REM stage from occurring. As a result, you wake up feeling irritable, depressed and may have difficulty concentrating. Some symptoms of hangovers may, in fact, be the direct result of REM deprivation.

Myth: Mild sleeping pills are safe to use for extended periods as long as I take them as directed.

Fact: Many sleep aids rob you of REM sleep, producing symptoms of REM deficiency. In addition, you run the risk of developing dependency and tolerance to these drugs if taken for prolonged periods of time.

Myth: If I suffer from insomnia, then I must have some deep-rooted psychological problem.

Fact: Insomnia may be an indicator of an underlying psychological dilemma. For the majority of the population, however, this simply isn't true. Insomnia, for many, is merely the result of faulty learning. When normal sleep resumes, the irritability and depression you may be experiencing quickly end.

Myth: Heavy snoring indicates deep and restful sleep.

Fact: Although heavy snoring may indicate deep sleep, it is not indicative of *restful* sleep. Heavy snoring, in fact, is frequently a symptom of sleep apnea, a serious and life-threatening disorder that is characterized by the inability to breathe adequately during sleep.

TYPES OF INSOMNIA

People who suffer from insomnia rarely feel robust. Although the negative effects of sleep deprivation are generally consistent from person to person, insomnia comes in a variety of forms and for a variety of reasons. As you read through the various types of insomnia, remember that some symptoms may overlap. You may, for example, have initial as well as terminal insomnia or experience multiple causes as the source of your sleeplessness.

Early Onset Insomnia

This particular type of insomnia begins in childhood and sometimes as early as infancy. For some people, this may be the result of a neurological imbalance. Some adults who suffer from insomnia report that they were diagnosed during childhood as hyperactive. Others may have experienced a learning disability such as dyslexia or a reading disorder. Reading disorders are due in part to an inability to integrate auditory and visual information, and may also be the result of an impaired ability to interpret spatial relations. To put it simply, reading-disordered refers to a child who had a difficult time learning how to read.

Other children may have had a biochemical disturbance which resulted in an abnormal sleep/wake pattern. Unfortunately, medical science has not been able to determine any laboratory tests that can detect these biochemical abnormalities. Clinical evidence suggests a possible biochemical basis for childhood onset insomnia and scientists are trying hard to find appropriate tests.

Most people, however, including those mentioned above, suffer from learned childhood onset insomnia. Many adults state that as children they had inconsistent sleeping patterns. As a result, a learned and reinforced pattern developed that they carried over into adulthood.

The following questionnaire will help you to determine when your pattern of disturbed sleeping began. You may need your parents' help to answer some of these questions.

Childhood Sleep History

1. As an infant, you were fretful, had feeding difficulties, and appeared to resist sleep.
   ❑ Yes   ❑ No

2. As a young child, you often stayed up past 9:00 p.m.
   ❑ Yes   ❑ No

3. You routinely fell asleep on the sofa or floor and were then carried to bed by a parent. You rarely fell asleep in your own crib or bed.
   ❑ Yes   ❑ No

4. Once in bed you had difficulty falling asleep.
   ❑ Yes   ❑ No

   A. You frequently awakened during the night.
   ❑ Yes   ❑ No

   B. You routinely awakened before 6:00 a.m. and were unable to return to sleep.
   ❑ Yes   ❑ No

5. You experienced frequent nightmares as a child.
   ❑ Yes   ❑ No

6. One or both parents suffered from insomnia.
   ❑ Yes   ❑ No

7. As a child, you learned to hide and suppress emotion.
   ❑ Yes   ❑ No

8. Your childhood sleeping conditions were so unsatisfactory (e.g. uncomfortable bed/noisy bedroom) that you had difficulty falling asleep or maintaining sleep.
   ❑ Yes   ❑ No

If you answer yes to two or more of the above statements, your sleep disturbance may be the result of learned childhood onset insomnia.

Learned Childhood Onset Insomnia

Being a new parent is a challenging job. Often, when a baby is difficult, parenting proves exhausting for both mother and father. Parents grow weary from the demands of a fretful infant. As a result, to quiet the demanding baby parents hold him more, and he receives more attention than the passive infant. The difficult infant quickly learns that this type of behavior allows him to gain control of his environment. Since sleeping patterns are just beginning to develop, parents lay the groundwork for the subsequent development of childhood sleep disturbances.

Whether due to permissive parenting or a fretful infancy and childhood, the development of poor sleep habits carries over into adulthood. Often a young child's sleep disturbance will abate during adolescence only to resurface later. If you have begun to experience insomnia during adulthood and have a positive response to the previous questionnaire, do not rule out learned early onset insomnia.

Nightmares can also be a factor in learning poor sleep habits during childhood. Frightening dreams often occur as a result of stress in a child's life. Often the stress passes, but the effects of nightmares may not. A child quickly learns to associate bad dreams with falling asleep. As a result, the child becomes afraid to fall asleep and, therefore, interprets it as something to avoid.

Sleeping disturbances can become easily established in a small child. All it may take is one to two weeks of consecutively bad dreams for a child to begin shunning sleep. Once this occurs, the fear of sleep begins to generalize. As a result, anytime this child experiences stress, sleep becomes something he consciously or unconsciously tries to avoid.

The adult insomniac unconsciously continues to associate stress with poor sleep. Although a conscious fear of nightmares may no longer exist, stress triggers the forgotten fears of childhood where stress produced nightmares and nightmares made sleep something unpleasant.

Modeling can also contribute to the development of insomnia. Children owe much of their approach toward living from behavior modeled by their parents. If a child hears a parent complain of chronic sleeplessness or sees this pattern in his primary caregivers, it quickly becomes acceptable behavior for the child. To compound the problem, a parent suffering from insomnia may be more tolerant of a child's pleas to stay up late. Often the sleep-deprived parent becomes more permissive simply because he or she may lack the energy to enforce rules. Since most children want to be like their parents, they emulate parental behavior and attitudes. Along with all the positive traits a child may assume, he also assumes less desirable ones, such as the tendency for insomnia. Negative patterns become easily learned and deeply ingrained.

The tendency to repress emotion is an additional problem common to many insomniacs. This is particularly true for those suffering from childhood onset insomnia. Poor sleepers frequently learn early in life to avoid emotional expression. Unfortunately, emotional release surfaces inappropriately in other areas.

Most of us are aware of the competent businessperson who develops ulcers. Few people realize, however, that insomnia is another avenue of emotional release for those who have difficulty expressing emotion. Insomnia caused by repression of emotion is frequently seen in adults who, as children, learned to suppress their discomfort and feelings. Men appear to suffer from insomnia more than women, partly because as little boys they may have received less approval for their emotional expression. As a result of avoiding emotional expression, depression frequently surfaces in the guise of physical disability such as headaches, hypertension, heart attacks, ulcers, or insomnia.

There is hope for repressors, however. If they can begin to verbalize minimally self-threatening emotion and gain confidence in doing so, they can gradually increase the depth of their self-expression. In time they may learn that mature expression of emotion enhances human relationships. Self-disclosure can reduce the level of depression and insomnia that frequently accompanies masking, and overall health can improve. These are all intervention techniques addressed in chapters 3 through 11, which focus specifically on therapeutic strategies for the remediation of insomnia and depression.

Adult Onset Insomnia

If your response was negative for childhood insomnia, you may be suffering from adult onset insomnia, such as persistent psychophysiologic insomnia or insomnia without objective findings. Both types of insomnia develop during adulthood and there is a strong correlation between the intensity of sleeplessness and stress. Although this stress is often psychological, it may be any source that taxes a person's resources such as pain, illness or drug addiction.

Persistent psychophysiologic insomnia is a sleep disturbance that assumes the characteristics of learned insomnia. It does not, however, have its origin in childhood. Typically, sleep researchers differentiate adult onset insomnia into three subtypes.

Although people suffering from each subtype share common symptoms of sleep deprivation, there are noted differences, as well:

A. Initial insomnia
   1. Delayed sleep onset
   2. Prone to general nervousness, anxiety or panic attacks
   3. Worries excessively
   4. Poor concentration
   5. Once asleep, may sleep very soundly
B. Interrupted insomnia
   1. Awakens intermittently throughout the night and has difficulty returning to sleep
   2. Often associated with medical complications such as chronic pain, respiratory and cardiac complications or diabetes (due to frequent nighttime urination)
   3. More prevalent in adults over 50
   4. Excessive caffeine intake or alcoholism
   5. Less likely to experience depression or anxiety
C. Terminal insomnia
   1. Awakens two to three hours before alarm
   2. Increased nightmares
   3. Shallow sleep
   4. Exaggerated rapid eye movement shortly after falling asleep
   5. Endogenous depression (depression due to a chemical imbalance within the brain)

By far the most dangerous insomnia is the interrupted type. This can be an indicator of serious, if not life-threatening medical complications. More critical, however, can be the effects of heart or lung disease. If you suffer from interrupted insomnia because of respiratory illness, you should avoid sleeping pills or tranquilizers. Sleeping medications and antianxiety agents relax respiratory muscles and reduce already deficient ventilation. This, in turn, creates greater oxygen deficiency which places an additional strain on your body. If you suspect that you may have a serious medical disorder you should avoid self-medication and seek prompt medical attention.

Adult onset insomnia has a wide range of causes. The following list indicates some of the more common problems that often contribute to the development of insomnia.

Medical

- Chronic pain caused by arthritis, illness, or injury
- Diabetes, resulting in frequent nighttime urination
- Cardiac or respiratory disease
- Premenstrual syndrome (PMS)
- Colitis, producing frequent diarrhea

Psychological

- Faulty learning in response to current stress
- Manic depression, resulting in a marked decrease in sleep
- Depression caused by a chemical imbalance
- Depression resulting from situational factors
- Post-traumatic stress disorder or PTSD (a reaction to a traumatic event)
- Anger, anxiety, or panic attacks

Chemical

- Diet pills, decongestants, caffeine, some antidepressants
- Dependencies such as alcohol and nicotine
- Reverse effects of alcohol and hypnotics (drugs with the intended purpose of inducing sleep)
- Major tranquilizers that can produce a state of restlessness and nervousness called akathesia

Insomnia without objective findings is an uncommon form of insomnia that causes added hardship for its victims. People who suffer from this type of insomnia complain of chronic sleeplessness. Family members, however, report that these individuals appear to sleep quite well. As a result, these insomniacs gain little support from others.

When these individuals enter Stage 2 sleep, however, they do not achieve the state of relaxation that the normal sleeper does. Instead, if awakened from Stage 2 sleep, they often give detailed accounts of their thoughts, suggesting that the normal thought-slowing process does not occur. Stage 2 accounts for three to five hours of a person's total sleep time. When restful sleep does not occur, therefore, sleep deficiency symptoms result. On a positive note, however, this type of insomnia responds as well to treatment as any other form of insomnia.

SLEEP LABORATORIES

The medical field has gained most of its knowledge about the sleep process through sleep laboratories, which are readily gaining recognition. Many major hospitals now offer these facilities to the public.

Typically, when an individual enters a sleep lab he or she follows a strict set of guidelines. An in-depth analysis of an individual's life style, medical history, and sleep patterns occurs before the actual sleep testing begins. Lab personnel provide questionnaires periodically throughout the testing procedure, before sleep and again after awakening.

When the lab technologists are ready, they instruct the patient to get into a laboratory bed within a comfortable homelike setting. Lab personnel then place electrodes strategically on the patient. The electrode placement is minimally intrusive and allows for considerable freedom of movement. Lab personnel instruct the client to fall asleep when ready.

The electrodes record certain sleep time activities of the patient. These recordings are called polysomnographs and usually include three standard measures. First, an electroencephalogram (EEG) monitors brain waves and allows for sleep stage scoring. Second, the electrodes record eye movement essential for determining and scoring REM sleep patterns. And finally, an electromyogram (EMG) reads muscle activity. Electrodes are placed on the skin over muscle groups and the EMG detects the amount of tension in these muscles. An electromyogram enables medical personnel to further study REM patterns and to look for additional sleep disorders, as well.

In addition to the polysomnograph, lab personnel scrutinize the client's sleeping behavior. Likewise, they check blood pressure, pulse, and temperature periodically. After completion of the polysomnograph, personnel awaken the client and study his or her waking behavior. The medical staff then analyze the test and observational data. From this, they devise a treatment plan and present the results to the client and his or her personal physician.

This brief explanation provides an overview of the basic methodology used within sleep laboratories. This is a complicated field, however, where sleep testing and analysis demand a highly trained medical team. Depending upon the needs of the client, therefore, a medical staff's testing guidelines vary dramatically.

Chapter 2
Common Causes of Insomnia

Physicians estimate that nearly 20 million Americans suffer from major depression at some time in their lives. If we include less severe forms of depression, the 20 million figure would likely triple. Mild depression is such a part of the fabric of American society that the actual prevalence would be impossible to calculate accurately.

Although there are numerous origins for insomnia from pain to rotating shift work, depression, anxiety, anger, and chemical dependency are the most common themes. Each of these four, singly, is sufficient to induce poor sleep; but often, instead, various combinations of these four factors contribute to the genesis of insomnia.

Unfortunately, once a condition of sleep deprivation occurs, it often serves to exacerbate the very condition that caused insomnia in the first place. Because of the complexity of the relationship of emotions and lifestyle to insomnia, people must expand their focus beyond their inability to sleep and asses the emotional and physical factors that contribute to and perpetuate their insomnia.

DEPRESSION

Often, insomnia is in itself an important indicator of underlying depression. Frequently, however, to avoid dealing with depression, sleep-deprived individuals focus on their insomnia instead. When people suffer from insomnia, they know they need sleep. When they're depressed, however, they frequently do not understand why they are unhappy. Others may feel unable to tackle their problems effectively. In either case, these people may unconsciously choose to avoid their emotional pain.

To determine whether your insomnia may be a mask for depression, we have constructed a simple test. By completing and scoring the mood awareness profile (MAP), you will be able to determine if you are suffering from depression—and to what extent. Some depressions may be severe, others may simply cause a person to feel unhappy. Whatever the case, a test such as this can create a new level of awareness. It can allow you to shift focus from insomnia to the real cause of your sleeplessness: depression.

MOOD AWARENESS PROFILE

As you complete the questionnaire, circle the appropriate number from 0 to 4 that reflects how you have been feeling for the past several weeks. If you suffer from long-term insomnia, however, answer according to how you have been feeling throughout the duration of your insomnia. If you have difficulty labeling your feelings, compare your current state of mind to how you believe a happy person feels. Leave no area unanswered.

	None	Rarely	Sometimes	Often	Always
Health worries	0	1	2	3	4
Guilt	0	1	2	3	4
Hopelessness	0	1	2	3	4
Anxiety	0	1	2	3	4
Loss of pleasure	0	1	2	3	4
Irritability	0	1	2	3	4
Boredom	0	1	2	3	4
Poor concentration	0	1	2	3	4
Withdrawn	0	1	2	3	4
Loneliness	0	1	2	3	4
Worthlessness	0	1	2	3	4
Fatigue	0	1	2	3	4
Change in appetite	0	1	2	3	4
Death wishes	0	1	2	3	4
Total each column:	0	_____	_____	_____	_____

Add column totals for final MAP score: _____

MAP interpretation: The highest you can score is 48; the lowest is 0. Like most people, however, your score will fall somewhere in between. The following chart shows the range for varying degrees of depression. The higher your total, the more severe your depression.

35 or above: Severe depression
25 to 34: Moderate depression
15 to 24: Mild depression
0 to 14: Normal mood fluctuation

You should retake the mood awareness profile every two weeks, so it serves as a barometer of the progress you are making as you practice the techniques in this book. As your depression and insomnia improve, your scores will decrease proportionally. Regardless of your score, however, if you feel that your life is unmanageable or you have suicidal thoughts, you should seek prompt intervention with a professional mental health specialist or through your local hospital. Most hospitals have a referral system that can link people to the appropriate community resources.

Types of Depression

The following classifications of depression often produce insomnia. The list is not all-inclusive, but it defines the types of depression people commonly experience who score above 24 on their MAP.

Major depression is a severe form of depression in which a person experiences profound despondency. Other symptoms include excessive fatigue, feelings of guilt and worthlessness, poor concentration, and loss of appetite. In addition, the individual's thought, speech, and movement are slowed and there is typically a decrease in sexual drive. It is not uncommon for the severely depressed person to become preoccupied with death and thoughts of suicide.

Major depression is frequently the result of a chemical imbalance within the brain. Often, those suffering from this type of depression cannot report any external stress in their lives that could be responsible for their depression. People suffering from this illness withdraw emotionally and often physically, and experience a diminished sense of pleasure from formerly enjoyable activities. Depression of this intensity profoundly affects a person's ability to relate to others, which often results in marital discord and job loss. Episodes of major depression often last six months or longer, and thoughts of suicide are common. Insomnia, or early morning awakening at least two hours earlier than scheduled wake-up time, may become routine. The average age of onset for major depression is in the late twenties. This type of depression is often hereditary, with blood relatives frequently experiencing depression, as well.

If you feel that you may fit into this category, you should seek immediate psychiatric consultation. If you have a history of depression within your family and do not have any negative situations in your life, your depression may be chemical in nature. Often, chemical imbalance (also known as endogynous) depression responds to proper medication with a marked improvement in mood and a more positive outlook toward life in general.

Dysthymic depression is a chronic form of depression lasting at least two years. A person suffers from some or all of the symptoms of major depression, but to a lesser degree. Suicidal thoughts may not be present. Social and occupational impairment are usually mild to moderate. Dysthymic depression typically has its onset during childhood, adolescence, or young adulthood. People suffering from this type of depression often appear gloomy, negative, and disinterested in life. Normal moods may occur, but they are brief and infrequent, rarely lasting longer than a few weeks. Some researchers suspect that a chemical imbalance may be present. It is more likely, however, that people suffering from this type of depression interpret their environment negatively, thus experiencing continual bad feelings.

Adjustment disorder occurs within a three-month period of an identifiable stressor (negative event). Typically, however, the individual's reaction is greater than what mental health professionals consider to be normal. The symptoms are similar to that of dysthymic depression, but the social and occupational impairment of the individual may be pronounced. When an adjustment disorder lasts longer than six months, however, doctors and psychologists usually reclassify it as dysthymic depression. Insomnia can be a major problem for those suffering from adjustment disorders.

Post-traumatic stress disorder is a reaction to an identifiable traumatic event such as war, a natural disaster, or a serious accident. This condition may be short-term or it can become chronic. Depression and anxiety follow the trauma and flashbacks (a sense of reliving the event) typically occur. These individuals startle easily and are often hyper-vigilant.

Sleep disturbances and nightmares, during which the person reproduces the traumatic event, are common. People suffering from this disorder often experience chronic tension, irritability, and an inability to tolerate noise.

There are other forms of depression whose complexity is beyond the scope of this book. To address them briefly would do the reader an injustice. Such depressions as the manic depressive types consist of mood shifts of psychotic proportions, which require an intense medical regimen maintained throughout the lifetime of the individual. The four categories we have discussed, however, are much more common, with insomnia frequently a common denominator among them all.

ANXIETY

Few cases of insomnia and depression (even milder forms) exist without the presence of considerable anxiety. Most depressed people feel underlying fear and tension. It is the combination of this fear and tension that creates a state of anxiety. The relationship between depression and anxiety is not totally clear, however. Some researchers believe that the basis of all depression is anxiety. When anxiety becomes chronic, depression becomes one's reaction to this anxiety. Others conclude that anxiety is a result of the debilitating symptoms of depression. In any event, it is unlikely that you will have one without the other.

General anxiety is as common among the American population as is mild depression. The symptoms so closely resemble that of depression, that it can be difficult to separate the two. Typically, anxiety-prone individuals are apprehensive and worried. They tend to over-react to and misinterpret the behavior of others. Anxious people have difficulty concentrating or making decisions and frequently question their own judgment. They often exhibit strained posture and overreact to noise or sudden interruption. Muscular tension is usually present, particularly in the neck and shoulders. Frequent urination, insomnia, and nightmares are common. Other notable symptoms include heart palpitations, breathlessness, and an increased pulse rate, all of which can overlap depression.

No matter how well their lives are going, anxious individuals always find something to worry about. This combination of excessive worrying and oversensitivity creates a state of constant apprehension and depression. When the anxiety prone climb into bed at night, they still can't turn it off. They remain overstimulated by obsessive worrying and often lie awake several hours before they finally fall asleep from sheer exhaustion. Once asleep, however, anxiety dreams take over, and nightmares of falling or being chased and not being able to run are common themes. As if this were not punishment enough, the anxious individual, because of underlying depression, often experiences terminal insomnia, as well.

People who are prone to developing chronic anxiety commonly assume one of four different personality types. Some may have difficulty being assertive; others may fear responsibility and independence. Interestingly, individuals who have difficulty complying or submitting to others frequently develop symptoms of anxiety. Trusting only in themselves, they assume others will fail them (possibly as their parents did when they were children). As a result, when forced to depend on, or comply with others, they become fearful. And, finally, there are anxious individuals who have learned to fear emotional intimacy. They crave intimacy with another, yet become anxious when it occurs, creating a state of pervasive anxiety as they continually search for intimacy and reject it the moment they find it.

The development of anxiety is complex. It would be incorrect to say that the four personality traits mentioned above are the sole causes of anxiety. Excessive stress or illness are but two of many other factors that can lead to anxiety. Nor will all people who have the above character traits develop symptoms of anxiety. If, however, a person experiences chronic anxiety without any negative life events, the above characteristics may be worth investigating.

One of the central features of most depression, and often the initial cause of anxiety, is loss. It may be the loss of a loved one, or a job, or the perceived loss of youth. The list goes on, and what may be meaningless to another may represent profound loss for you. It is also important to remember that when loss occurs, change results. Not only do you mourn the loss of a significant factor in your life, but you must adjust to a different world—a world that is suddenly without a familiar and important aspect of your daily routine. This is a demanding task for most of us and, as a result, anxiety becomes one of the snags frequently experienced. You may begin to feel overwhelmed, and your thinking is likely to become distorted and negative.

Unfortunately, depressed, anxious individuals often take a passive stance. They believe they are victims of depression and there is little they can do to alter their condition. A depressed person frequently feels inadequate and incapable of meeting what she perceives to be excessive demands from her environment. She views the people who are most important to her as unsupporting and considers her future as bleak and unpromising. This attitude, in turn, spreads and permeates other areas of her life, as well. What often begins as mild depression escalates into a more severe mood disturbance, preventing her from engaging in new and positive behaviors and attitudes.

If you scored at or above 27 on your MAP, it is likely that your insomnia is a result of depression. Scores lower than 27 suggest that the depression you are experiencing may be a symptom of sleep deprivation. Although insomnia can cause mild depression, it is usually a life filled with stress (which you feel powerless to change) that is the real cause of your insomnia.

ANGER

Anger is a necessary emotion in the human repertoire of expression. When maturely and appropriately expressed, anger can serve to motivate and protect us. Frequently, however, we are not mature in our expression and conflict results. Unhealthy conflict not only affects our relationships with others, but produces internal conflict, as well.

People frequently and inappropriately suppress their anger. This anger eventually surfaces, however, and expresses itself through a variety of symptoms that many people do not recognize as anger. If you feel depressed and get little enjoyment out of life, unrecognized anger may be the cause. If you suffer from chronic insomnia, anger can, once again, be the culprit. Frequent headaches and ulcers can also be indicators of suppressed anger.

To help you recognize your own anger and the negative power this emotion can have on you, we have provided a simple questionnaire. The results may give you some added insight into your own behavior, and allow you to see the consequences of anger that is not maturely expressed.

Anger Awareness Survey

1. Do you adamantly deny having feelings of anger?
   ❑ Yes   ❑ No

   Denial is often an indicator that you feel anger that is deep and intense, which you feel uncomfortable recognizing. By feeling intense anger, you fear that you may lose control over what you feel incapable of managing. Strong denial is often a protective mechanism that allows you to avoid the fear that results from strong emotion.

2. When you do express anger, is it usually directed at someone or something seen as less powerful than you?
   ❑ Yes   ❑ No

   For example, do you explode in anger at your children for some minor infraction, yell at the dog, or kick the garbage pail? This is usually what happens when intense anger is felt toward a person or situation that you believe is more powerful than you. As a result, you direct your anger inappropriately.

3. Are you a procrastinator?
   ❏ Yes   ❏ No

Procrastination is often a form of rebellion in which a person, angry and dissatisfied with life, tries to strike back by not cooperating. He rebels against his responsibilities by avoiding what life and other people demand that he do.

4. Are you accident prone?
   ❏ Yes   ❏ No

Frequent injuries are often a product of anger turned inward. You direct your anger toward yourself because you perceive yourself as a less powerful and threatening target than the real source of your anger. If you frequently hurt yourself, your accidents may not be accidental at all.

5. Do you have frequent headaches?
   ❏ Yes   ❏ No

Anger makes people tense. Although you may not recognize your anger, your body will respond to the negative emotional climate. The result is tight muscles that give rise to tension headaches. Tension is often a product of frustration, and people who are frustrated are people who are angry.

6. Do you compulsively overeat?
   ❏ Yes   ❏ No

Overeating can be an aggressive act of unconsciously stuffing angry feelings. Again, this act often represents anger directed toward self. Unlike the accident prone, however, the compulsive overeater gains the reward of temporary relief from unwanted feelings. She may feel frustrated in response to a life filled with chaotic emotion. Since the compulsive overeater feels incapable of dealing effectively with her emotions, her response may be one of anger. In her attempt to avoid dealing with this anger, the cycle of binge eating continues.

7. Do you have feelings of hopelessness?
   ❑ Yes   ❑ No

Feelings of hopelessness frequently represent anger in its most passive form. Hopeless, depressed individuals, like those in question 1, often deny being angry.

8. Do you forget to follow through on promises you've made to others?
   ❑ Yes   ❑ No

This is a passive-aggressive form of anger. Frequent forgetting, or absentmindedness, may appear innocent, but it is often an unconscious expression of suppressed anger toward others. Uncomfortable with overt expressions of anger, these individuals passively act out their rage. Their forgetfulness often thwarts plans others have made, thereby unconsciously satisfying an angry person's need for retaliation.

9. Do you cry easily when you feel stressed?
   ❑ Yes   ❑ No

Crying is a response that people commonly interpret as meekness. In actuality, however, it is frequently an expression of anger that feels powerless to defend itself.

If you answered yes to any of the above questions, it's time for you to begin practicing self-observation. If unexpressed or misdirected anger is an underlying problem for you, it just may be responsible for many of your sleepless nights.

Anger is an emotion common to all, and as children we expressed it openly. If your brother took a toy from you, chances are you hit him. When you didn't get your way you may have had a temper tantrum. As we grow into adults, however, through parental and societal intervention, most of us learn to control our expression of anger. Nevertheless, this does not assure that we learn how to manage this emotion effectively. As a result, anger may surface in a variety of unhealthy ways. Some may develop insomnia, others may develop a cynical outlook toward life, and others may develop into violent and dangerous human beings. No matter how it manifests itself, when anger is not dealt with appropriately it disrupts lives.

Even though most of us cannot afford to express our anger openly (such as telling a hateful boss where to go), we must not deny it. Admitting to and recognizing anger in ourselves does not mean we have to actively express it. In fact, active expression is rarely in our own best interest. What it does mean, however, is that we do not deny or mask this emotion. It is the act of denying and masking anger that results in its misdirected expression or physical and psychological problems. Recognizing the source of the anger is often the first step toward effective problem solving.

In most cases, the way you vent your anger is a learned process. Anger is an emotion common to all, but the way you express anger today depends upon how you were encouraged to express anger as a child.

To gain mastery over the expression of this emotion, you must first recognize it. For some people this is easily done. Others, however, such as the procrastinator or compulsive overeater, may have a more difficult time.

Once you can identify your anger, you must begin channeling this emotion constructively. As long as you continue to act out your rage physically, argumentatively, or through destructive hidden modes such as those mentioned above, you cannot learn to manage your anger effectively.

Popular opinion suggests you can harmlessly vent your anger toward inanimate objects, such as, for example, hitting a pillow or kicking your tire. We believe, however, that this type of behavior serves only to escalate your hostility—not resolve it.

When you become angry, certain physiological responses occur. Your adrenal glands (one resting atop each kidney) secrete epinephrine and norepinephrine, your body's arousal hormones. These two hormones produce an increase in your blood pressure, heart rate, and breathing. In addition, muscle tension and perspiration increase. This release of arousal hormones creates a very negative internal environment for managing strong emotion. Activities such as yelling, throwing objects, or even hitting a pillow serve only to increase the production of these stimulating hormones, thereby intensifying your anger. The greater the amount of epinephrine and norepinephrine in your system, the more agitated, violent, or self-destructive you are likely to become. You may believe that you are harmlessly redirecting your anger, but your adrenal glands treat anger as anger, no matter where you direct it. Instead of redirecting anger, your goal should be to neutralize it.

Redirecting, denying, or swallowing anger often results in psychosomatic illnesses such as ulcers, arthritis, and high blood pressure. To avoid the ill-effects that mismanaged anger and its hormonal stimulation can produce, you must recognize your anger, then channel it constructively. Constructive expression of anger can take many forms. It may be physical, such as jogging, lifting weights, or playing tennis. Or it may be through creative expression, including activities such as writing, playing the piano, drawing, or painting. You must interrupt your anger by engaging in any activity that you find pleasurable and entertaining.

Constructive and enjoyable activities such as these can block your body's excessive production of epinephrine and no-repinephrine. This allows you to use up the excess arousal hormones circulating within your system. As a result, you calm down and gain a more realistic perspective of your situation. It does more than this, however, because as you engage in personally pleasurable activities, your body releases another chemical. This one, unlike excess epinephrine and norepinephrine, has a healing effect upon the body.

Produced within the brain is the chemical called endorphin. Considered to be the human body's natural pain killer, endorphin has additional benefits, as well. Scientists have discovered that minute quantities of endorphin are 50 times as powerful as similar amounts of morphine. In addition to this, research suggests that endorphin release produces an increased sense of calm and well-being (endorphin is the natural chemical associated with runner's high). Although its primary purpose is to reduce pain, its added properties are exactly what an angry person needs to reduce his or her level of arousal.

One of the fastest and most effective means of reducing excessive levels of arousal hormones (and increasing endorphin production) is aerobic exercise. Any activity resulting in an increased need for oxygen can quickly reduce the negative effects caused by anger. And it does so more quickly than less active methods of release. However, if you are over 35 years old, or have an existing illness, you should get clearance from your doctor before engaging in strenuous exercise.

If you have pushed your anger beneath your conscious level of awareness, and it surfaces through frequent headaches, insomnia, compulsive overeating, or some other misdirected form, the same methodology applies. First recognize your anger and then take positive action.

By engaging in 20 to 30 minutes of daily exercise (or creative expression), four or five times per week, you can reduce the production of excessive arousal hormones, and thus begin the road to mastery of inappropriate anger. Overcoming anger, whether overt or repressed, is a gradual process. However, as you begin to release negative energy in a positive direction, you may find that both mental and physical health improve. You may realize over time that as your rage and irritability become more manageable, you can cope realistically and effectively with your emotional response to life.

The techniques provided in chapters 3 through 11 offer direction in helping you deal more effectively with your emotions. Whether your insomnia is a product of depression, anxiety, or anger, these guidelines will enable you to channel your emotions in a more positive direction. The result is often a better night's sleep and a more productive approach toward living.

CHEMICAL DEPENDENCY

Can you imagine that your sleeping pills, pain medication, or tranquilizers may be responsible for your insomnia? Well, they can be, and two interrelated phenomenon play a part in keeping you from a sound and well-rested slumber.

The first factor in the chemical dependency/sleep equation is the development of tolerance. Like hands developing calluses from hard physical work or skin tanning in an attempt to protect itself from ultraviolet rays, your body tries to defend itself from the ingestion of foreign chemicals. This mechanism of tolerance is the primary responsibility of your liver. It is within the cells of the liver that an enzyme called lysozyme is produced. This particular enzyme is responsible for destroying foreign chemicals circulating within the blood. When, for example, alcohol or other drugs are introduced to the body, lysozyme goes to work and begins to disintegrate these chemicals. The higher the drug level, the more lysozyme the liver must produce.

Unfortunately, lysozyme does not go away. The new cells that subsequently form within the liver and take the place of older ones have higher than normal levels of lysozyme. In other words, chronic users of drugs and alcohol have developed a high drug-burning furnace which results in a permanent tolerance to these chemicals. Narcotic addicts, for example, have developed such a high tolerance that the amount of drugs they can take in one day could kill 10 nonaddicted people with normal lysozyme levels.

The liver begins developing a tolerance to drugs, including tranquilizers and sleeping pills, within a two- to four-week period. Unfortunately, the human body's attempt to protect itself results in severe damage to the liver.

Just as high levels of lysozyme damage the body, a second phenomenon, called the compensating build-up factor, contributes to the development of insomnia. Simply put, the nervous system seeks to maintain a relatively constant level of sensitivity that becomes compromised when you take drugs such as tranquilizers that dull your senses. Although your headache may go away, your nerves calm, or you may fall asleep, this isn't a natural desensitizing process.

In your body's attempt to maintain its regular level of sensitivity, it begins to counterattack the drugs. By the time you have been taking this drug for two or three weeks, your nervous system is overcompensating. Thus, your brain increases its effort to stimulate itself in direct proportion to the strength of the desensitizing drug. As a result, the brain's natural sensitivity level increases. Therefore, you would have to take increasingly larger doses of these medications to achieve the same effect the drug initially produced. As a result, the brain becomes overly sensitive to other stimuli such as noise or minor stressors. Unfortunately, this increased sensitivity worsens the very condition you took the drug for in the first place.

Worse yet, if you abruptly stop your medication after long-term use, you are at risk of developing seizures. When a person stops taking medication the confused nervous system responds as if the person took the drug anyway. Since there is no chemical in the body to counter excessive stimulation, the nervous system virtually vibrates from ordinary stimuli. The reticular activating system loses its ability to screen effectively and becomes acutely sensitive to even minor background stimuli, such as a ticking clock or the sounds of passing traffic. As a result, a person experiences hyperirritability, and noise and minor stressors are magnified out of proportion. In some cases this excessive sensitivity can result in hallucinations or the sensation of crawling skin or seizures.

Even if you don't have sleeping difficulties you can develop insomnia if you begin taking sleeping pills on a regular basis, and do not increase the dose. This same principle holds true whether you take pain pills or tranquilizers. If you don't have a problem and you start taking these medications, you will develop one.

To stop these medications abruptly after taking them daily for periods longer than two or three weeks can be unsafe. We recommend, therefore, that anyone taking large amounts of medication for a prolonged period speak with his or her doctor about a drug-reduction regimen to wean him- or herself gradually off the medication. Your situation may be less severe, but the principle remains the same. If you want to increase the severity of your insomnia, nervousness, or pain, take the prescribed medications for these conditions. We are not saying that these medications cannot be appropriate for short-term use. We can almost guarantee, however, that long-term use will intensify the very problem that prompted you to take the drug in the first place.

DRUGS AND INSOMNIA

Western societies are acutely drug oriented. Without giving it much thought, people ingest numerous drugs and chemicals throughout their lives. Their days begin with caffeine and continue interspersed with alcohol, nicotine, aspirin, and artificial sweeteners. Every meal eaten is laden with chemicals—some harmless, some not so harmless. It is little wonder, then, that a chemically oriented society such as the United States would view sleeping medications as effective and innocuous alternatives to sleeplessness.

Although we recommend natural methods to promote sleep, we want you to be aware of the critical effects that sleeping medications can have. The following list provides practical information on the general classifications of drugs that people use for sleep. Although drug names differ they may fall into the same classification and will produce similar effects within the body.

Most of the drugs used for sleep produce a change in mood and behavior by depressing the central nervous system. Their primary effect is on the firing rate of the neurons within the brain. Although some drugs increase the rate of neural firing, such as caffeine and amphetamines, sleeping pills inhibit the firing rate of brain cells. Drugs that stimulate or inhibit the central nervous system are called psychotropics.

Although the list of this group of drugs is virtually infinite, it focuses on the group of psychotropics that millions of people use to fall asleep at night.

Barbiturates: Derived from barbituric acid, barbiturates provide heavy sedation and relief from insomnia and pain. Unfortunately, prolonged or excessive use of barbiturates leads to addiction and personality deterioration. Withdrawal from these drugs must be physician supervised, as people may suffer convulsions or death by abrupt cessation of the drug. Because of the dangers associated with barbiturates, physicians rarely prescribe them today. Some common barbiturates include phenobarbital, Amytal, Seconal, and Nembutal.

Narcotics: Narcotics are derivatives of the opium poppy; however, synthetic narcotics are available today, as well. This classification of drug effectively relieves pain and coughing and promotes sedation. Morphine, Demerol, Percodan, and codeine are examples of narcotics. Although addiction to narcotics under a medically supervised regimen is rare, physicians must monitor their patients for excessive sedation, nausea, vomiting, and constipation. All narcotics, however, are highly addictive and severe withdrawal symptoms from these drugs sometimes prove fatal.

Benzodiazepines: Benzodiazepines are among the most frequently prescribed medications in the United States, with physicians writing an estimated 68 million prescriptions per year.

Benzodiazepines fall into two subgroups: minor tranquilizers and hypnotics. The minor tranquilizers include, but are not limited to:

- Valium
- Librium
- Centrax
- Xanax
- Ativan
- Serax

Since these drugs can also induce sleep, they deserve special consideration. Although their intended purpose is to produce quick relaxation and a reduction in anxiety, this may be all the insomniac needs to promote sound and restful sleep. Unfortunately, they lose their effectiveness after several weeks, producing an ever-increasing tolerance to the drug. As a result, anxiety and nervousness begin to resurface and increase if a person doesn't increase the dose of the drug.

Abrupt withdrawal of benzodiazepines can produce muscle cramps, nausea and vomiting, and tremors and convulsions. Therefore, when a person withdraws from these drugs he must do so slowly. These complications can begin to occur after 24 hours if a person reduces his regular intake by one-half or more. Unfortunately, a person continues at risk for up to six weeks after he stops taking the medication.

Although hypnotics have chemical properties similar to minor tranquilizers, their intended purpose is to produce sleep. They act upon the central nervous system by reducing alertness and increasing reflex time. They also depress respiration, which is dangerous for those with sleep apnea. The most widely used hypnotics include Dalmane, Restoril, and Halcion.

Halcion is an extremely potent hypnotic that produces a powerful and fast effect. Not only does it put people to sleep quickly, it wears off approximately four hours after a person falls asleep. This allows a person to achieve normal sleep the last half of the night and awaken feeling well rested. For those new to the drug or the elderly, however, Halcion may cause some daytime sedation and confusion. Restoril, on the other hand, induces sleep more slowly. Its effect lasts six to eight hours and reportedly causes less daytime sedation. Dalmane is similar to Restoril, but it can produce a hungover feeling well into the following day.

Ambien, a relatively new hypnotic, is chemically unrelated to benzodiazepines and has fewer side effects. It produces no daytime grogginess or hangover and does not interfere with deep sleep stages 3 and 4. It has a rapid onset like Halcion and should be taken at bedtime and not before. Like all hypnotics, Ambien is intended for short term therapy since prolonged use can produce tolerance and dependence.

Unfortunately, prolonged use of any of the benzodiazepines results in tolerance and dependence. And prolonged use constitutes anything over a few weeks! The dangers, however, exceed even drug addiction. When taken on a daily basis, benzodiazepines can accumulate in the body and produce a buildup of toxic substances. Toxicity can reach a critical level within one week. Should this buildup occur and a person consume alcohol or take other medications at the same time, a fatal interaction may result. Research also indicates that some benzodiazepines taken during the first trimester of pregnancy may cause congenital abnormalities in infants.

Over-the-counter sleep aids: These represent any drugs that can be bought without a prescription. Over-the-counter (OTC) medications that people use to promote sleep usually contain antihistamines as their main ingredient. Although these drugs are often effective in initially inducing sleep, drug tolerance happens quickly and the human body requires increasingly larger doses to feel sleepy. In addition, antihistamines can cause dizziness, blurred vision, ringing in the ears, and nausea. In fact, anyone suffering from asthma, prostate enlargement, or glaucoma should avoid antihistamines altogether. Since a tolerance to these medications quickly develops, people often increase the amount they take, believing this is a harmless practice since they can buy these drugs without a prescription. They mistakenly think no prescription means no danger. Unfortunately, this type of thinking can result in self-poisoning.

Sleeping medications offer a quick fix for insomnia but they do not offer a real solution. Not only do they cause tolerance and addiction, but they also produce shallow sleep by interfering with the natural sleep cycles. Interrupted sleep cycles produce increased nighttime awakening which inevitably leads to an increase in daytime sleepiness and irritability.

In addition, benzodiazepines can remain within your body for two to three days after you stop taking them. Unfortunately, dangerous and sometimes fatal drug interactions can continue to occur if you take another medication during this time. Therefore, if for any reason, you need to take a sleep-promoting medication, speak with your physician about the effects of long-term use. In addition, you should request a medication insert from your pharmacist listing drug interactions and precautions.

Withdrawal Techniques

Suspect that you have developed a tolerance to sleep-promoting medications if your prescribed dose is no longer effective. If you have developed a tolerance you must gradually reduce your intake of the drug, while concurrently applying the management methods outlined in this book.

We recommend that you speak with your doctor about reducing your intake of medication. However, a typical method of weaning a person off of benzodiazepines is as follows. If, for example, a person has been taking 30 milligram capsules of Dalmane, his physician will prescribe a one month's supply of 55, 15 milligram capsules. Every third day he will take one 15 milligram capsule instead of the usual 30 milligram dose. Unfortunately, he must tolerate the minor sleep deprivation that will initially occur with this regimen. The second month he will alternate daily between 15 milligrams and 30 milligrams. The third month, he will take 15 milligrams for two days and 30 milligrams every third day. By the fourth month, he will have reduced his intake to 15 milligrams per night. Finally, he will abstain from taking any medication once a week for two weeks, then twice a week for the next two weeks. He will then proceed to every other day, and the following two weeks he will stop taking the medication altogether.

It is a difficult task to free yourself from the holds of a habit-forming drug. For those of you who do manage to withdraw from sleeping medications, however, you must follow a lifetime regimen of positive living. If you don't take preventive measures, it becomes too easy to fall back into bad habits at the first sign of stress.

If the reason you take sleeping pills is because of underlying psychological factors, you need to be honest with yourself and seek professional help. By seeking help, you are taking the first step toward a higher quality of living. It is easy for many people to admit they have high blood pressure and seek an expert's opinion. So why not seek an expert for depression, nervousness, and anxiety? Mental health professionals can't fix the problems in a person's life, but they can introduce positive coping skills, thereby reducing the need for drugs.

Antidepressants: Antidepressants increase the amount of specific chemical messengers within the brain that are deficient in depressed individuals. They also appear to produce an increase in the chemicals needed for sleep. These medications have no habit-forming properties, nor do people develop a tolerance to them. The sedative effects of antidepressants appear very quickly, usually within the first day. The positive impact upon depression, however, may take two weeks or longer for an individual to notice. If your insomnia is a product of depression and anxiety, certain antidepressants also have excellent hypnotic effects. Three particular antidepressants are especially beneficial for insomnia caused by depression:

- Surmontil
- Desyrel
- Pamelor

Many people who suffer from insomnia have underlying and subtle depression they may not even be aware of. To detect hidden depression, a physician should assess you by asking specific questions about your mental health and lifestyle (see MAP). If your doctor thinks it is appropriate, she will prescribe an antidepressant.

Many insomniacs suffering from depression who are dependent upon sleeping medications often get profound relief with the help of antidepressants. When a person takes antidepressants, he or she reduces the need for habit-forming hypnotics. In addition, if taken at bedtime, withdrawal from hypnotics proceeds much faster. We recommend supervision from a psychiatrist, however, to monitor possible drug interactions and side effects.

When people are addicted to drugs and not just experiencing tolerance, however, they develop many more side effects toward non-habit-forming drugs like antidepressants. Possibly due to their subconscious desire, the side effects provide an excuse to stop taking the replacement and return to the original drug. This is completely involuntary on the part of the individual, and is the addicted mind's attempt to maintain the addiction.

Because of the dangers associated with sleeping pills, we recommend a drug-free approach to sleep management. By committing to follow the methods addressed in this book, you can avoid the inevitable negative results that sleeping pills invariably produce.

Chapter 3
Think Yourself to a Better Night's Sleep

This chapter focuses on self-management techniques for the effective treatment of insomnia. It begins with the active process of therapy, focusing on cognitive, behavioral, and psychoanalytical methods of self-management. This chapter includes the development of self-observation and analytical skills, focusing on methods to lessen the negative thinking patterns that often produce insomnia.

These terms may sound unfamiliar to you now. You can, however, learn to use these techniques for effective self-therapy and alleviation of insomnia. We have taken a holistic approach to the management of insomnia, meaning we look at the various roles that the mind, body, and spirit play in sleep disorders, and how the body can be treated as a whole to promote better sleep. Since some forms of insomnia are the result of unmanaged emotions, this book takes an in-depth approach to solving the conflicts these emotions can cause.

Before you can successfully master the skills for effective lifestyle change, however, you must begin by changing the negative way you think about yourself and the world. The depressed person suffers from illogical and distorted thought patterns, which is usually the result of learning irrational beliefs from childhood experiences. The person may have seen negative coping behaviors in his parents and tuned into their attitudes. By observing, learning, and repeating, families pass negative coping styles and attitudes from generation to generation. The individual has learned unrealistic beliefs resulting in his expecting and demanding too much from self, others, and the world.

A good example of negative thinking is seen in many adult children of alcoholics (ACOA). Often, as children, ACOA's experience abuse, deprivation, rejection, and neglect. As these children mature into adulthood, they react toward the world in the same manner as they reacted toward their alcoholic parent. They are frequently angry, mistrustful, and lack the ability to be open with others. Often, these individuals develop the same thought patterns as the chemically dependent parent. Addiction in adult children of alcoholics is common with a tendency to think and behave like their alcoholic parent.

In the face of stress, many adults who have been the product of faulty parenting assume a self-defeating, self-devaluing, and negative attitude. Unfortunately, this negativity provides fertile ground for the development of depression and insomnia.

In addition to childhood experiences, the adult must deal with all of the stressful complexities of life in the 1990s. From financial difficulties to disrupted relationships, from physical illness to the loss of loved ones through death, the factors contributing to the genesis of depression are many. Some situations we can change; others we must accept. In either event, however, we can alter our coping strategies to help us live more effectively.

FEELING BRAIN VERSUS RATIONAL BRAIN

We store our perception of ourselves and the world in two portions of the brain that constantly interact with one another. This interaction results in either positive or negative attitudes and emotion. It is this interaction process that is the target of the cognitive therapeutic techniques discussed throughout the remainder of this chapter.

Current understanding of the anatomy of the brain suggests connecting pathways exist between the frontal lobe (the reasoning and judgment center) and the limbic system. The limbic system is the seat of many emotions and is a relatively primitive portion of the human brain.

The frontal lobe, or reasoning brain (RB), dictates realistic appraisals of people and situations. Through the interconnecting pathways, the reasoning brain interacts with the limbic system, or feeling brain (FB). This is a normal process and necessary for good mental health.

When there is an imbalance between this interaction, however, certain personality traits can develop. For example, people who appear rigid and emotionally constricted often have a low level of FB interaction. On the other hand, those with a restricted RB often respond much more emotionally toward life than the average person. As a result, these individuals are more likely to develop depression, anxiety, and other negative emotional responses. It may be the FB that produces emotion, but it is the job of the RB to turn this raw emotion into nondestructive, logical expression.

There is constant interaction between these two portions of the brain, but the limbic system always seeks dominance. The FB has complete access to the thought processes of the RB and tries to distort the RB's decision-making abilities. As a result, rational thinking becomes negative and irrational. Consequently, a person begins to feel that he lacks the ability to change his distorted thinking, which has become governed by emotion. The FB knows the RB's weak points and attempts to exploit them, using them to the FB's own benefit. The FB seeks instant gratification, desiring any shortcut to pleasure—including inappropriate emotional release. The FB can confuse the RB with overemotionalism. It uses these emotions to manipulate not only the RB, but other people, as well. It will go to any length to get its own way, often creating, for example, arguments with others that we may later regret.

Although the FB is very influential, we cannot underestimate the power of the RB. When properly trained, the RB can greatly influence the FB. A person can learn to think realistically and avoid many of the pitfalls that can lead to depression and negative relationships with others.

It is possible, very simply, to create a healthy balance between FB and RB by challenging overemotionalism with logical thought. The FB will try to trick your RB into thinking that your emotions are actually thoughts and not feelings. By practicing the following exercises, you can learn to replace negative feelings with realistic thought. You can learn to develop the ability to confront depressing emotion. You need to ask yourself, Where does this thought really come from? Is my FB trying to take over; have I stopped using my logical and intellectual resources to assess this situation? Am I, instead, allowing emotion to rule and distort my life? Our FB is a master of disguise. It often overpowers our RB and instead of logical thinking, we become charged with emotion. Our RB is confused into believing that what we feel is thought.

If we think an action is wrong, we feel bad about engaging in that activity. For example, if you think it is wrong to steal, your guilty feeling if you were to steal would be appropriate. This is the process of the RB logically influencing the FB. If, on the other hand, you think you must be a perfect parent and then feel bad because you're not, you have allowed your FB irrational control of your RB. Feeling brain thought is not logical thought, but instead is often an erroneous manipulation of fact. However, we buy into it anyway. If you want to have control of your feelings instead of your feelings having power over you, you must learn how to think rationally. Change the way you think, and you can change the way you feel. It works—quickly.

As we grow into adults, we allow our FB to control our lives. FB emotions become automatic pilots—often guiding us in directions that are not in our own best interest. We believe we are powerless to change because we think we are the victims of our feelings.

RULES TO LIVE BY

We all live by a set of unarticulated rules. These rules make up our value system, contribute to our moral fabric, and provide us with the framework for which we judge ourselves and others. We learn these rules through the attitudes and actions of others. We are taught these unwritten rules by family, our educational system, and society at large.

Many of these rules are distorted by the imaginative and literal interpretation of the young child's mind. We outgrow many of these distorted viewpoints, or thought errors, but by no means all of them. As children, we heard so many times that we had better be good little girls and boys that we learned to believe in the need for perfection. Although we can never attain this state, many of us never stop trying. Our irrational feeling brain makes us feel guilty or worthless if we don't continue to strive for this illusive state of perfection.

As we become adults, many of us maintain these illogical assumptions and as a result depression often follows. These irrational thoughts, maintained by the feeling brain, continue even in the face of contradictory evidence. The individual becomes so entangled in self-defeating attitudes that he or she selectively views the world as harmful and filters out positive information. These rules, developed in childhood, and often in the context of a negative or stressful event, become our distorted thinking pattern as adults and our perspective toward every situation. This type of locked mind-set increases our vulnerability and predisposition toward depression. And, once depressed, our distorted thinking serves to maintain this depression. This creates a vicious cycle of increasing depression and expanding control of our irrational FB to include a larger and larger range of situations.

The following table provides a list of the most frequently used thought errors. These thought errors are the basis for much of our distorted thinking and become the unwritten rules we live by.

Table 1: Thought Errors

1. *All-knowing:* On the basis of your negative feelings, you predict others' reactions to you in negative terms not based on fact.

2. *Guardian angel:* You see yourself as responsible for the reactions of others to their environment.

3. *Twisters:* You distort a situation based upon your interpretation without any facts to back it up.

4. *Emotional error:* You accept your feelings as facts.

5. *Victimization, "Poor me" attitude:* Usually sandwiched between self-pity and frustration, producing bitterness and depression based upon focusing on the past—a means to avoid responsibility for your present and future.

6. *Microscoping:* You look for a minor detail in a situation and exaggerate its significance, inferring negative consequences.

7. *Negating options:* Getting stuck in emotional quicksand, ruling out options for change.

8. *Perfectionistic thinking:* If you don't live up to your super demands 100 percent, you view yourself as a total failure.

9. *Positive filter:* The filter rules out positive factors with a total focus on negative aspects that serve to enhance and maintain a negative view of self and the world.

10. *Word extremes:* Making statements in negative absolute terms: I am stupid; I hate myself; I am a total failure; I always disappoint others; I never do anything right.

11. *No mole hill policy:* Everything has mountains of feelings attached to it.

To gain effective self-management skills, you must begin by determining your own unwritten rules. Once you are able to do this, you should be able to differentiate your feelings from rational thought. This is a very important first step. By developing the ability to separate feeling from thought, you can stop trying to force feelings to change. This is an impossible task unless you take a chemical that temporarily masks your feelings of fear and anxiety. You can put these negative and frightening feelings on a back shelf until the alcohol or pills wear off, but you can't get rid of them until you get rid of what is causing them. You can cover them up and bury them—but you can't make them go away.

We express many of these unwritten rules automatically without thinking. These automatic thoughts, usually the product of our feeling brain, become accepted as fact and go unchallenged. We recommend that you begin keeping a daily log of your automatic thought responses. This should be done for a two-week period on the charts provided in appendix 1. Table 2 provides an example of the technique you should use in filling out your forms. This overview shows you the automatic FB responses that are most common in depressed individuals. When you fill out your own chart note the thoughts that make you feel depressed. These thoughts will most likely repeat themselves. You may find that new ones emerge and others may lessen. A pattern, however, will begin to emerge in which you can determine what your negative thought distortions are. Move slowly, as you begin to challenge emotion that has been passing for thought. You must be patient and thorough. Focus on one problem area a week (but be flexible with yourself—if you need two weeks, take two). You should begin to notice an improvement in your mood if you follow the instructions outlined in the remainder of this chapter. Remember: Automatic thoughts are usually gut feelings. The very nature of that statement shows its error!

Table 2: Automatic Thought Form

Automatic thought: I hate this job. I've been here 10 years and no one has ever told me that I've done a good job. It makes me so angry.

Distorted thoughts: Word extremes like "hate" or "no one." *No one* has *ever* told me.

Feeling: Anger and hate and resentment (often feelings are the verbs in the sentences).

Rational thinking: Maybe my boss hasn't told me I have done a good job, but he certainly has showed me that he appreciates me. I have had several promotions and some substantial raises. Besides, I feel I do a good job and I take pride in that.

Thought error: Filtered out positive information and viewed only negative factors to enhance a negative point. Watch for word extremes—always suspect some inaccuracy if they are used for negative purposes. Extremes rarely occur. In addition, I view my negative emotions as facts. Remember, they aren't facts, they are merely feelings and highly subject to error!

When you notice that you are engaging in automatic thought, use the trigger words: rational thought. Silently or out loud, repeat these words three times. This serves to interrupt your irrational thought cycle, allowing you to shift your focus from negative to positive, enabling you to distance yourself temporarily from your feelings. Now, challenge your thinking. Is that gut feeling really true? Step outside of yourself. Look at the situation as if it were another person's problem. If the same automatic thoughts have occurred four or five times throughout your two-week recording period, you can bet this pattern is a contributing factor to your level of depression.

When you finish your two-week log, review it by spending a week focusing on determining any emerging patterns. Every time your automatic thought surfaces, challenge it with your thought error and rational thought response. It takes effort. You can't give into the automatic feelings that trigger your irrational thoughts and make you miserable. Refuse to entertain these automatic feelings. Let them serve only to trigger rational thought. If you do this for one to two weeks you will find that your feelings begin to respond to what your rational thoughts are programming.

In just a short period of time, your feeling brain will become more mature, the feelings much less stress inducing: this will be your first step in self-managing what you thought you were powerless to control. It feels good not to get upset over things. It feels peaceful and pleasant and enables you to focus on the more enjoyable aspects of living. It takes work, but if your depression falls into the mild to moderate range, you can learn to lower your MAP scores if you diligently practice these cognitive techniques.

If you have difficulty analyzing your automatic thoughts, try applying the following questions. These will often clarify a clouded issue:

1. In my situation what is fact and what is merely belief?
2. a What is the evidence that supports my automatic feeling brain thinking?
   b What is the evidence that negates my automatic feeling brain thoughts?
3. Are there any other explanations for my circumstances?

4. If I were happy, how would I perceive this situation?
5. What's the worst that could happen—realistically—and how do I deal with it?

And remember, most depressed people treat their automatic irrational thoughts as if they are facts—laws written in stone which can never be broken. The automatic thoughts you have are merely *your* perception of the world (and possibly your parents). It happens to be your particular view at any given time—but it's a constricted and depressed view that is ready for change. As depression becomes increasingly severe, remember that automatic feeling brain thinking becomes less and less related to reality.

JOAN'S STORY: USING YOUR THOUGHT JOURNAL

Joan, employed as a full-time secretary and a part-time student by night, has been feeling somewhat overwhelmed and depressed lately. On this particular day she overslept, rushed to get ready for work, and, taking a last-minute glance in the mirror, told herself she looked horrible. Arriving at work, tired from studying too late the night before, she felt quiet and not in the mood for socializing with co-workers. Her job seemed tedious this day and incredibly dull. She knew her boss didn't approve of the report she had submitted, and, when she finally left for school, her frame of mind was hardly conducive to taking an exam. By the time she arrived home, she had managed to convince herself that she had failed her test and that she was too stupid to do anything right. If Joan began her day feeling depressed, by day's end she was surely feeling worse!

Let's analyze Joan's automatic (FB) thoughts in the thought journal format and see if she could not have avoided much of her unhappy feelings had she employed rational thinking instead.

Automatic thoughts: I look horrible and I feel so ugly.
Distorted thoughts: Looking horrible.
Feelings: Feel ugly and poor self-image.
Rational thinking: I have been letting myself look a little sloppy lately. I am not ugly though—as a matter of fact, I feel pretty good about myself when I fix myself up a little bit. Maybe it's time for a new hairstyle.
Thought errors: Ruling out options for change. If I don't like something about myself, I do have the power to change it. I get stuck in emotional quicksand and lose sight of the fact that I have choices and options for change.

Automatic thoughts: I don't see how anyone could like me. I embarrass myself, I am so dull.

Distorted thoughts: I am totally unlikeable and incredibly dull.

Feelings: Worthlessness and embarrassment for self.

Rational thinking: I happen to have quite a few friends who seek out my company, and I do have numerous interests. No one else ever responds to me as if I'm boring—besides, I'm just tired today and I'm getting that confused with feeling negative about myself.

Thought errors: Drawing conclusions that are not based on fact. I have been rationalizing feelings—I have allowed feeling worthless to become a fact. It is only my feeling and that certainly does not make it a hardened fact.

Automatic thoughts: I am so disgusted with myself. If only I had my act together and I could go to school full-time, I could graduate much sooner and get out of this dead-end job.

Distorted thoughts: I am so disgusted with myself. *If only* I could go to school full-time.

Feelings: Worthlessness and self-pity.

Rational thinking: I may be in a dead-end job, but I am doing something about it. I wish I could move faster than I am, but my grades would suffer and most probably my health if I attempted to work and go to school full-time. I have always wanted to go to school and I am finally doing something about it. I have taken charge and that makes me feel pretty good about myself.

Thought errors: Ignoring the positives and only recognizing the negatives. I employ unrealistic self-expectations, demanding from myself what I would never expect from another. I must be aware of "if only" statements, as they usually are sandwiched between self-pity and frustration—the combination of which produces bitterness and resentment. Fortunately, "if only's" are rarely based upon fact.

Automatic thoughts: I know my boss didn't approve of the report I submitted.

Distorted thoughts: I know my boss didn't approve.

Feelings: Anger and low self-esteem.

Rational thinking: As far as my boss's attitude about me? Well, he has always treated me with respect and frequently gives me assignments that are above and beyond the role of a secretary, because he knows this job is rather boring for me. He must think that I am capable. He has never disapproved of my work in the past, so it is unlikely that he will now, either. If he does—well, it will be the first time. Pretty good record, but then I am competent!

Thought errors: Believing that I have the ability to read another's mind and assuming that their thoughts are negative, even though the evidence points to the contrary.

Automatic thoughts: I know that I failed my exam. I am so stupid—I just can't do anything right.

Distorted thoughts: I know that I failed and am stupid and can do nothing right.

Feelings: Worthlessness and stupidity.

Rational thinking: I don't know how I did on the exam. I have never failed a test yet and, even if I do, which is very unlikely, it will not have that great an impact on my overall grade. Besides, if I fail a test it, doesn't mean I'm stupid; it means I haven't prepared adequately.

Thought errors: All-knowing—I don't have the results of the test back yet, so it is merely prediction on my part—not fact. I employ all-or-nothing thinking—I take a single situation and base my entire self-worth on it. If I don't achieve 100 percent, then I have failed. I must beware of "word extremes," where I state things in absolute terms. Absolutes are usually rare events.

You can use this case study and Joan's thought journal to assist you in interpretation of your own automatic thoughts. A more complete chart of thought errors is provided in table 3. Analyze your illogical thoughts and search for the flaws that trigger feelings of unhappiness and insecurity. Initially, however, your feelings are not going to "believe" your rational thinking process. Your emotions have been conditioned for too long to respond to your negative automatic thoughts. Keep repeating the rational thoughts every time an irrational automatic thought comes into your mind. Often, the reconditioning process will begin to take effect within one to two weeks for any particular feeling you want to improve. Your feeling brain begins to respond to the logical thoughts—and you begin to feel happier, more mature, and better equipped to deal effectively with yourself and others.

By following the thought journal format you can begin to break down your depression into manageable parts. List the automatic thoughts and prioritize them, from used most often to least often. Become aware of your style of thought. By becoming familiar with your distorted response to yourself and your environment, you can begin to gain insight into the causal factors of your depression.

Don't demand perfection from yourself. You may stumble occasionally and forget to challenge your thoughts. The key is not perfection, but persistence. If on a bad day you have 100 distorted thoughts and you only challenge 10 of them you're still making progress. Be patient with yourself—and don't give up. It gets easier.

When you begin your thought journal, do not try to change your thinking while logging your two weeks' worth of thoughts.

You want an accurate account of the distortions you employ—not a modified or edited version. At the completion of your journal, begin reviewing it and note the merging patterns.

As you construct your hierarchy of distorted thoughts, we recommend that you begin challenging those thoughts employed least often. These thought patterns are least ingrained, and easier to challenge. This will give you confidence to move on to frequently used, and thus more difficult, thought patterns to change.

As you progress from least to most difficult you should begin noticing a graduate improvement in your mood. As your depression lessens, you will have more energy to challenge the more frequently used automatic thoughts at the top of your list.

The first week you may find your mind resists change. You may conveniently forget to challenge your thoughts or even have episodes of "What's the use?" thinking. Your automatic thoughts are possessive and your feeling brain will try to trick you into avoiding change. Again, be patient and begin by challenging "What's the use?" thinking as your first automatic thought response. As your self-monitoring skills increase, you will gain momentum and the process of self-therapy will become easier.

This revised way of thinking can enable you to become more in touch with yourself. You may begin to realize that your automatic thoughts are governed by your feeling brain and are not a product of rational thinking. This is also an appropriate time to begin developing insight into the reasons why this negative thinking occurs. Ask yourself: Was this what I learned from my parents? If not, what significant person in my life have a copied this behavior from? Who do I remind myself of when I think and act this way? This type of introspection is valuable not only for the depressed, but for adult children of alcoholics and co-dependents as well. As you complete your thought journal, jot down possible causes of your negative thinking under the "Origin of Thought" section.

Chapter 4
Use Mind Power Effectively

We cannot will ourselves to fall asleep in the same manner that we decide to stay awake. The desire to maintain a state of wakefulness requires active energy and we cannot use this same type of energy to fall asleep. The relaxation and sleep state require a process of letting go of energy—not harnessing it to try and force oneself to sleep. The only thing this accomplishes is maintaining a high state of wakefulness. Unfortunately, for many people the desperate determination to fall asleep results in an unending saga of sleepless nights.

This chapter addresses the insomniac's hypersensitivity to her environment and offers destimulating techniques and rules that promote restful sleep. These methods can reduce the sleep-related anxieties that often develop into full-blown sleep phobias. By focusing on your cognitive ways, you can apply these guidelines and lay the foundation for successful sleep management.

Direct (Active) Control/Indirect (Passive) Control
Direct control is the power that helps us with the voluntary functioning of our minds and bodies. We can direct these voluntary functions toward creative expression in art, or the physical movement of our muscles in dance, or the energy employed while at work or driving the car. These are all examples of direct energy. This is a voluntary, activating energy and the same type that the insomniac uses when trying to fall asleep. Using this energetic determination is very effective in maintaining a state of wakefulness, but useless for sleep.

In addition to direct control, but rarely used by Western society, is passive control. This is the indirect process that enables us to ease gently into sleep, without battle and minus all active energy. This is a passive approach that you can learn in much the same way that you have learned to approach life with a constant need for direct control.

Sleep, unlike wakefulness, is an involuntary process, functioning much as the digestive or cardiovascular system. Sleep is necessary for survival and like all biological functions, occurs without effort on a normal sleeper's part. However, as with any physiological system, sleep can go awry in much the same way that a person develops an ulcer or high blood pressure. Frequently, the cause is often the result of a life filled with anxiety and unresolved stress. And, as you cannot actively will your ulcer to heal or blood pressure to go down, you cannot force sleep. It is in this perspective that indirect control becomes an important instrument to promote sleep. Although we lack active control over involuntary processes, we do have the ability, though often untrained, to influence biological functioning in a passive but positive manner.

Most of us have not only heard of, but fully accept, the concept of psychosomatic illness. Although we lack active control over our cardiovascular and digestive systems, we realize there exist certain connections between our bodies and minds. Most of us know someone who has developed an ulcer or colitis or possibly high blood pressure after prolonged periods of stress. We accept this connection readily. We believe in the negative impact the mind can have on the body—often without question. And yet, how many people openly accept the ability of this same mind to heal its body? If we can effect negative consequences to our overall health, why can't we heal ourselves as well? Through proper learning techniques you can transform this negative energy and redirect it into constructive healing and health.

Mind/body medicine has begun to be a topic of serious study by many scientists. Although considered quackery in the recent past, Western scientists are now employing serious effort in an attempt to unravel the mysteries of mind over body. They have studied masters of yoga from Eastern cultures and have acknowledged the positive impact of their beliefs with regard to mind/body integration.

How does a person will himself to develop heart disease, high blood pressure, insomnia, or ulcers? These negative body states are often a result of an indirect process—the passive control gone awry. We can redirect this negative and indirect process that causes involuntary malfunctions such as hives, nausea, and high pressure, and train it to promote health and well-being. This training process is what the remainder of the book is about. With motivation, practice, and the combining of techniques addressed throughout this book, you too, can develop the skill to promote restful sleep and a healthier tomorrow.

MANAGEMENT OF INSOMNIA

We have already talked about the reticular activating system and how it promotes a state of alertness and wakefulness. To fall asleep, however, this portion of the brain must passively destimulate, allowing the sleep-promoting portion of the brain to take over. As the reticular activating system begins this process, a person enters Stage 1 sleep, a twilight state between wakefulness and actual sleep. At this stage the sleep-stimulating portions of the brain become dominant and a person enters Stage 2 sleep, and the cyclic process begins.

With the insomniac, however, the normal passive destimulation response does not occur. With the poor sleeper, the reticular activating system becomes more easily and quickly aroused than with the normal sleeper. For example, the mere act of watching the clock at night can induce stress in the insomniac and produce excess stimulation. Every time she looks at the clock, she once again arouses her reticular activating system. Unfortunately, each activation can continue 10 to 15 minutes before the destimulation process begins again. Because the insomniac is so easily aroused by normally innocuous stimuli, it becomes easy to see how a state of chronic sleeplessness is maintained.

The area of sleep promotion focuses on the destimulation process, whether it's to fall asleep initially or, after waking, to return to sleep. With all forms of insomnia, two situations appear to occur with regard to the destimulation phase:

1. The individual becomes excessively concerned about his need for sleep and, as a result, tries to force himself to fall asleep. This, in turn, is sufficient stimuli to maintain a state of arousal.

2. The person unconsciously learns not to destimulate. A stressful period in a person's life may trigger an episode of sleeplessness which in turn becomes generalized to the very state of sleep itself. Thus, insomnia may persist long after an individual resolves the crisis in his or her life.

The remainder of this chapter focuses on techniques that will help you reduce your hypersensitivity to your environment and your negatively learned sleep habit.

A frequent trait of insomniacs is the racing mind syndrome. If you're like many other poor sleepers, you find that as you climb into bed at night, you drag your troubles with you. Instead of drifting off into a quiet, peaceful sleep, your mind refuses to let go of all the irritations of your day. Forty-five minutes later, you're still awake, problems remain unsolved, and you rest assured that you will have another sleepless night.

One effective alternative is to set aside 30 minutes per evening for an intense worry session. Since worrying has a randomness about it that only creates more mental chaos, we recommend that you buy a notebook and devote your worry session to the concrete task of putting pen to paper. This serves a twofold purpose: It allows you to organize your problems instead of getting lost in the chaos created by worried thought, and, in addition, you can challenge the automatic thoughts that are the foundation of much of your worry. You can use the same format as the thought journal included in appendix 1.

We recommend that you do this at the end of your day, before bedtime. When you close the cover on your journal, allow your problems to stay there, symbolically separated from you until the following day.

One little-known fact is that good sleepers awaken 5 to 15 times every night. They think some nonthreatening thought and drift off to sleep again, unaware they had even awakened. Poor sleepers, however, who invariably fear insomnia, are immediately aroused. They interpret awakening as a stressful event and respond to turning a normal five-second arousal into a two-hour catastrophe.

If you are one of these interrupted sleepers who, once awake, becomes immediately aroused, do not stay in bed. Initial and terminal insomniacs should employ this technique, as well. Get up and leave your bedroom. It becomes tempting to stay in bed and ruminate about your inability to sleep or to turn on your light and read. Your only accomplishment, however, is the development of a strong association between sleeplessness and your bedroom. Go to another area of the house and engage in some quiet activity until you once again feel sleepy.

The negative association that develops between sleep and your bedroom can do much to perpetuate your insomnia. Regardless of how tired you may feel, if sleeplessness persists over 20 minutes—get up and leave your bedroom. If you can follow through consistently for a two-week period, this often proves sufficient to extinguish the association between lack of sleep and your bedroom.

This simple technique produces excellent results—but only if performed consistently for at least two weeks and thereafter anytime sleeplessness occurs. The problem for most insomniacs, however, is that they fall into the trap of trying to force sleep. To many troubled insomniacs, the very act of getting up represents defeat. Beware of this kind of thinking. It will maintain your state of insomnia and prevent you from following through for any type of program completion.

If you go to bed and do not fall asleep within 20 minutes or you continue wide-eyed for 10 minutes if you awaken during the night, make yourself get up. It becomes tempting to continue lying there, because although your mind may be racing, your body feels exhausted. The aggravation of getting up becomes one more trial in a difficult day.

If you're serious about putting an end to your insomnia, however, you must make a total commitment to this program. Anything short of 100 percent will not produce results. If you get up 90 percent of the time, the other 10 percent is sufficient reinforcement to maintain the negative association between sleeplessness and your bedroom. If you believe that you may have difficulty being consistent with this exercise, you may prefer focusing on the passive techniques addressed in chapters 5 through 7. You can always return to this method at a later date.

Often, insomniacs report that they have trouble sleeping during their stressful work week, but on weekends they sleep like babies. Upon further investigation, it turns out that during the week they go to bed at 11:00 p.m. but on Friday and Saturday may stay up until 1:00 or 2:00 a.m. This appears harmless enough, and for the normal sleeper it is. For the insomniac, however, this presumably innocuous pattern, coupled with job stress, is a trigger that can maintain their sleep disturbance. By throwing off her work schedule by as little as two to three hours on weekends, the insomniac manages to disrupt and confuse her delicate natural rhythm and thus perpetuate her sleeplessness. When the new week rolls around, the hypersensitive insomniac cannot respond to the demand to go to sleep two to three hours earlier than the day before.

It is of paramount importance for the poor sleeper to maintain a consistent bedtime. This consistency establishes a natural rhythm that promotes sleep and reduces any confusion to the easily aroused sleep system of the insomniac. Some individuals opt to go to bed a little later during the week, so they do not feel they are shortchanging themselves on weekends. If you opt to sleep later on weekends, make sure you do not stay in bed longer than two hours beyond the time you normally get up on workday mornings. This may sound like a rather boring way to treat your days off. For the insomniac, however, a routine sleep schedule becomes as important to help control sleeplessness as hypertensive medication is for those with high blood pressure.

The three techniques explained here are to be done in conjunction with automatic thought challengers and biofeedback exercises. If this is done, you will have achieved sufficient behavioral and cognitive modification to ensure the attainment of a good night's sleep.

It should be clear by this time that you must make major lifestyle changes if insomnia is to be laid to rest. If you allow approximately three months to work through the techniques outlined in this book, you can achieve effective lifestyle modification to attain sleep mastery.

Chapter 5
The Power in Resignation

We have discussed concrete, active measures for management of depression, anger and insomnia. Unlike these active approaches, however, resignation is a passive process of letting go. A process whereby you release—not control—the energy that results in anxiety and hyper-arousal. Unfortunately, most Americans have not learned this lesson. Instead, Western society is a hard driving, action-oriented culture; its members have accomplished more in the past 100 years than all previous eras combined. Despite this advancement, however, society has exacted a price. Treatment for stress and stress-related illnesses has reached epidemic proportions.

Over the past several decades, people have become accustomed to working hard and getting results. For many of us, it's not enough to have control over our own lives. We feel a responsibility to exert this same influence on others as well. We become emotionally involved in the outcome not only of our own lives, but in those of other significant people—our children, parents, co-workers, or friends. We assume responsibility for our world and all who come into contact with it. We assume this responsibility not only for life-altering situations, but for everyday, minor concerns as well.

For most of us, our own problems are enough to cause mental fatigue. It's little wonder we can't sleep at night when we assume responsibility for the problems of relatives, friends, and peers. Not only does your mind race about your daughter's impending divorce, but your spouse's snoring isn't conducive to sleep, either. It is in these matters that you can begin to learn the art of resignation. As you become proficient in this area, you can progress toward more complex matters. Not only will you sleep better to the sounds of snoring, dripping faucets, and traffic, but you will learn to resign control in more serious matters, as well. By letting go of your need for control, you can develop a more reasonable and rational approach toward the circumstances in your life.

Resignation and acceptance are synonymous. By letting go and voluntarily giving up control, you can accept situations as they are and not as they should be. For example, let's take a particularly annoying example—snoring.

Due to the emotional response toward a snoring roommate, many lose sight that snoring is an involuntary process on the snorer's part. The snorer can't help it. We lie there listening, wide-eyed in the dark, with resentment building. It's not the snoring roommate that is the problem; rather, it is our decision to become emotional that keeps us awake. The first step in resignation is to accept that you are powerless over another's snoring. When you become upset over your roommate's snoring (or worrisome thoughts, the barking dog, or a host of other concerns), you stimulate the release of epinephrine and norepinephrine, which merely serves to intensify your state of wakefulness.

Often people respond to this line of reasoning by saying, "But I have no control over my anger. I just get so angry I feel myself boiling inside." Well, as humans, we do have control over much of our anger. We control it in countless ways throughout our day, and do so without so much as even giving ourselves credit for having done so. How many times do we respond to situations by thinking: It's not worth it, I'm not going to upset myself. And yet we all have troublesome areas in our lives that we just can't let go of.

So, if you have trouble resigning with acceptance, there remains the option of resignation with neutrality. In this mental frame of mind, you exercise your ability to bypass emotionalism and assess your reaction. You do not focus on the stimuli that is causing your reaction. You can learn to step outside of your emotional response and enter a state of neutrality. You can accomplish this in much the same way that a good reporter objectively reports the news—stating the facts as he sees them, avoiding any type of emotional reaction toward the story.

This state of objectivity and neutrality enables you to realize that your reaction is an overreaction. You may begin to see that you have had certain negative feelings in general toward this person and have felt unable to express those feelings honestly. As a result, you take a backdoor approach, an easier and far less effective approach to these negative emotions. You may have difficulty being assertive, or it may be that the real issue is too sensitive to address directly. Instead, you focus on something of little consequence into which you can vent your anger. However, dealing with negative emotion in an indirect manner frequently backfires. By not dealing with the real issues, you have created additional problems. You focus on an involuntary behavior such as snoring and allow it to create added hostility.

The true act of resignation involves more than just letting go. It would be wonderful if it were that easy. However, it's not. You must enter a state of emotional neutrality where you put your emotion aside, if only briefly, to objectively observe your reaction. True resignation allows you to become more in touch with your feelings. You may realize, for example, that it's really not the snoring that bothers you, but some negative feelings toward the snoring person. After all, you can probably remember when you just started dating your partner and the snoring was a reassuring reminder that the love of your life was there by your side! This is true with many types of stimuli. For example, many sleep wonderfully to the sounds of a pounding surf, yet complain of sleeplessness from the noise of a dripping faucet. As you can see, the impact of positive and negative emotions associated with the waves or dripping faucet or snoring becomes obvious. To take this one step further, if you were paid 20 dollars an hour for every hour your roommate snored, would it be annoying to you then? Although the example we just gave is laughable, it brings home the point that it is a person's attitude, and not the stimuli, that is often the real cause of sleeplessness.

Resignation is not always taking the easy way out, nor is it a passive response of acceptance with futility. It is a positive acceptance of life, where you change what you can and accept what you cannot change. In our example of a snoring spouse, accepting the snoring is not possible until you step outside of your emotional reaction. To accept the snoring as something you *can't* change, you must be frank and begin dealing with issues within the relationship that you *can* change. Until you determine the real source of your resentment behind your displaced anger, resignation will not be possible. As you begin to recognize that you may have deeply buried the real issues, you may find that snoring really isn't the problem at all.

This carries over in many situations, whether it is the dripping faucet, the thunderstorm, the sound of traffic, or the barking dog. Resignation becomes possible after entering the neutral zone and excavating for real issues (and few of us come up empty-handed). We may find that we perceive a stimuli as obnoxious because we have anger and frustration that is being misdirected. It is much easier to get angry with your neighbor's dog than discuss communication problems with your spouse.

How many of us, when relaxed and comfortable, can fall asleep to the murder and mayhem being committed on television? Or, as we mentioned earlier, when young and in love, accept our lover's snoring as a sign that he is really only human after all—thank heaven! And what about the time a co-worker asked if the storm last night kept us awake, and we had to ask, "What storm?" The point being, when some nighttime sound is a real nuisance, chances are it isn't the sound alone, but some other issues that we would prefer *not* to deal with! The focus of this book is not to help you resolve the particular stressors in your life. We want to help you get a good night's sleep—to put an end to your insomnia. As is often the case, however, insomnia is often a product of unresolved conflict of which you may or may not be aware.

If you do not have any underlying conflicts, but nocturnal noise continues to keep you awake, it will be easier for you to develop the skill of resignation than the person who uses environmental noise as a transfer source for anger ventilation. It is impossible to block noise completely—certainly not in the same manner that you can turn your head and stop looking at an object. Hearing is, in fact, a safety mechanism that protects us from harm by keeping us alert and prepared for fight or flight in the face of impending danger.

If you can't sleep due to environmental noise or your racing thoughts are keeping you awake, we guarantee becoming emotional over it will make your insomnia worse! You may get angry with your auto mechanic because your car isn't ready and it may speed him up, but it will not work with insomnia! The insomniac climbs into bed at night, the negative programming kicks into action, and the futile attempt to force sleep begins. This creates a negative feedback loop, working in a cycle to maintain insomnia. You tell yourself you're not going to stay awake even though you *know* you will! You create a no-win situation for yourself and one that is certainly not conducive to sleep.

You must begin to understand that environmental noise is not as much of a problem as your attitude and approach is toward that noise. You attempt to force sleep by trying to ignore sounds or by demanding that your mind turns itself off. This, unfortunately, only creates greater neuronal excitability, which in turn results in frustration, anxiety, and a perpetual state of wakefulness. For example, by trying to force your mind to block a particular thought, you find, instead, it is the only thought you can think about. This is a situation in which your dynamic energy works against you.

To prove this point, let's perform a simple experiment. For the next 60 seconds think of anything you want, except an elephant. Put the book down and try it.

How did you do? You probably did rather poorly. No matter how hard you tried, you just couldn't get rid of that annoying image: elephant. This is exactly what happens when you lie in bed at night, mind racing, trying to control your thoughts in order to force sleep. You watch the minutes and hours pass, knowing that you are only going to get five hours sleep if you fall asleep *right now.* This becomes your elephant.

When you do go to bed, the first concrete step you can take to eliminate this elephant is to stop trying to force yourself not to think. Allow the thoughts to come. Become an audience to your thinking, as if you are listening to a radio and unable to turn it off. You must admit that you are powerless over these thoughts and accept that they are there. Choose not to get emotional over them, as the emotional stimulation does more to keep you awake than the thoughts themselves. Accept the thoughts as you have accepted that snow is white and fish swim. If the content of your thoughts is disturbing to you, visualize a large stop sign. Picture this in your mind for 5 to 10 seconds and then shift the focus of your thinking to something pleasant. Thought changing using this technique becomes easier with practice. We will discuss this process of visualization in depth in chapter six.

It is also important that you try to limit positional changes. The more you move about, the more you continue to stimulate your reticular activating system. This prevents the sleep-promoting center in your brain from gaining dominance and producing the relaxation necessary for sleep. Accept that you may not find a position that is immediately comfortable. Just lie as quietly as you can. After a relatively short time, you will begin to feel restless.

It is in this area of trying to force sleep that phobias toward insomnia develop. The insomniac feels that she should get the same immediate response when she turns the lights out that she gets when she turns the key in the ignition of her car. Anything less than immediate sleep indicates malfunction and produces severe anxiety. Reluctant to experience any degree of sleeplessness, the phobic insomniac is at risk to develop dependency upon sleeping medications.

Often, phobia-prone insomniacs are self-demanding, self-critical, and action-oriented people who believe that anything less than perfection represents a loss of control and failure. They frequently report bedtime anxiety symptoms such as tingling hands or feet, rapid heartbeat, shortness of breath, or a sensation of chilliness or nausea. If you experience any of these symptoms, however, we recommend you visit your doctor to rule out possible physical complications.

Often, insomniacs have control in so many areas of their lives that they expect they should be able to exert this same dynamic approach toward sleep. The more elusive sleep, the more important this physiological function becomes in the mind of the phobic insomniac. In fact, sleep often becomes the primary focus of his or her life.

By practicing and applying the process of resignation, you will no longer have to fear climbing into bed at night and not being able to sleep. There are no magic pills, however. You have to become involved in and accept responsibility for your own therapy. We provide the guidance and direction, but you must provide the means of transportation and the energy to reach your destination.

To be effective in the self-management of insomnia, you have one fundamental requirement: unconditional self-acceptance. While practicing your techniques, it is paramount that you avoid all self-condemnation. It is okay for you to evaluate your progress, but you must not rate your worth as a human being based upon this progress. The two are mutually exclusive! As you practice the techniques in this book, it is not an option for you to engage in self-deprecating thought. The 30 minutes or so you spend daily working through your exercises is 30 minutes that *you* spend being kind to *you*. Be proud of yourself—you're making positive effort for positive change.

Chapter 6
Using Biofeedback to Calm Yourself to Sleep

In this chapter, we provide you with private biofeedback instruction. Our step-by-step training format enables you to achieve the same benefits as those achieved with expensive electronic gadgetry. And all for the mere cost of this book!

Typically, biofeedback uses monitoring equipment to provide information on involuntary processes such as muscle tone, blood pressure, skin temperature, pulse, or brain wave patterns. Ordinarily, since the body does not receive any feedback on a conscious level from these involuntary systems, it has very little control over them. When the body finds a way to receive information from some of these systems, however, it can train the mind to influence these involuntary functions.

Scientists have developed a variety of equipment aimed at providing clients with continuous information about the involuntary functioning of their bodies. Two such types of biofeedback devices that are popular today are the electromyogram (EMG), and alpha wave monitors.

The EMG reflects muscle tension through the aid of electrodes attached to the arms, legs, and facial area. These sensors are particularly sensitive to the electrical activity within the muscles. The electrical impulses received by these sensors are then fed into a monitor that translates this information into a continuous beeping sound. The beeping sound enables the client to become aware of the degree of his or her muscle tension. The faster the beep, the faster the muscles firing rate and the greater the degree of overall tension. Scientists have determined that a direct correlation exists between muscle tension and states of stress and anxiety. Therefore, the slowing of the beeping sound indicates not only increased relaxation in the muscles, but a reduced level in one's overall perception of stress, as well.

The alpha wave method of biofeedback also employs the use of electrodes attached to the skin. Technicians place these sensors on the forehead and monitor certain brain wave activities. This is a painless procedure that enables the client to discern the level of alpha or beta brain wave activity. Alpha waves register 8 to 12 Hertz and reflect a calm, relaxed mental state. Beta waves at 13 to 26 Hertz represent states of alertness, vigilance, and tension. The overall goal is to increase the production of alpha waves, thus increasing one's sense of relaxation and calm.

These are just two of the many methods of biofeedback measurement that are currently in use. With any biofeedback method, however, the basic approach remains the same. Through the use of monitoring equipment, the individual becomes alerted that tension levels are high. Through a step-by-step process this person develops the ability to alter her negative state of mind and lower body tension. She learns to make an association between her positive mental action and the signals of the monitoring equipment that registers increasing levels of relaxation. Thus, people successfully learn to use relaxation techniques to lower stress levels, promote sleep, and reduce pain. Biofeedback is the process of learning mind over body techniques, a process in which a person can increase body awareness and learn to let go of the determined need for perfection.

You, however, are going to bypass the expensive equipment and use your own body sensations as your biofeedback tool. Costly electronic gadgetry in biofeedback clinics is fun to use and certainly serves its purpose. It does little good, however, when you are restless and unable to sleep in your own bed or stuck in rush hour traffic. The purpose of biofeedback is to increase your level of awareness, an awareness that you need to control the tension that keeps you from feeling your best and even prevents you from sleeping at night.

The equipment signals a person as to how well he or she is doing with the techniques, but by simply using body signals you can do the same. Unfortunately, many people who receive instruction with monitoring devices do not receive the psychological and physical tools needed to use these techniques once they return home. Without these, a person often lacks confidence when trying to practice the techniques outside of the clinic setting. And when a person lacks confidence, he is one step away from discouragement. Therefore, you will achieve greater certainty and competency in your biofeedback skills if you learn to interpret your own body signals and not those of machinery. We believe this is a far more effective means to help you manage the stressful areas in your life.

LET'S BEGIN

We are going to take you through six biofeedback sessions, such as those done in expensive treatment centers and hospitals. It is our recommendation that you undertake no more than two sessions per week, practicing each until you become proficient. In our last session, we troubleshoot, discussing possible obstacles you may encounter and how to deal effectively with these problems. Many people begin to feel more relaxed after the first few practice sessions. To achieve these positive results, however, you must make a commitment to follow through with the program. We recommend that you practice a *minimum* of 20 to 30 minutes daily, *at least* four days per week, preferably five. *When* you practice is up to you. Some people prefer bedtime, others the morning, others after work. We have found, however, that most insomniacs benefit with a bedtime routine.

Breathing Technique—Session Number 1
Most healthy people take breathing for granted, rarely reflecting on the marvelous mechanism that it is. The life-giving oxygen that we breathe in and exhale as carbon dioxide waste must exist in a delicate balance if we are to maintain a state of health. Frequently, however, when we are angry, anxious, experiencing pain, or feeling overtired, we begin to lose our synchronized breathing pattern. When this happens, an imbalance develops in our ratio of oxygen to carbon dioxide. This change in breathing is often so slight it may pass by unnoticed. However, even a slight change in respiration is enough to affect your body chemistry.

This imbalance in the ratio of oxygen to carbon dioxide can produce a variety of symptoms. Symptoms range from a constriction in blood vessels within the skin to a fall in blood pressure, shortness of breath, lightheadedness, a tingling sensation in hands or feet, muscle spasms in one's extremities, and a general sense of weakness. Although sleep-deficiency symptoms may not be severe enough to result in actual physical impairment, the breathing pattern is such that a mild and chronic dioxide imbalance results.

This brings us to the deep-breathing technique. People often lack interest in this particular area because they do not understand the mechanism behind it. When asked why they believe deep breathing can be effective many respond vaguely with, "Well, it's slow and steady and it just makes you calm down." This type of statement shows a lack of understanding. If that was all there was to deep breathing, we wouldn't bother either—but there's more than that. Many women, when properly trained, accomplish the entire act of childbirth by using the deep breathing technique alone! Not only can it work, but it does so exceedingly well. The problem is that most people do not spend enough time learning and practicing proper technique so that it is effective in time of need. It does work, however. Ask any woman who has delivered a child naturally!

Deep breathing is more than a psychological catharsis or a time out mechanism. When done properly, it produces a calming effect by synchronizing your breathing and using maximum lung capacity. As a result, your carbon dioxide and oxygen resume a normal ratio. When practiced routinely, deep breathing can help restore feelings of well-being by reducing the side effects that improper breathing can cause. You can use deep breathing to promote sleep, to calm feelings of nervousness or anxiety, and to alleviate nausea and headaches. In other words, deep breathing comes in handy any time you need to feel better.

You can get started by assuming a comfortable position. Perhaps you prefer a favorite chair or your bed or the floor and a soft pillow. It's up to you—wherever you feel the most relaxed. When you practice, your legs should remain uncrossed with your arms positioned loosely at your side.

Now let's begin. I want you to breathe in very slowly through your nose to the count of six (one-thousand-one, one-thousand-two, etc.) and completely fill your lungs. Then hold your breath briefly to the count of four . . . and now slowly exhale, through your mouth once again to the count of six, making sure you completely empty your lungs. This process should not be uncomfortable for you. You can adjust the rate of your breathing if the six-four-six method is too difficult. You can begin with four-three-four and gradually increase your length if you feel more comfortable with this pattern. Repeat this slow, deliberate process three more times. Make sure that as you breathe in, you push out your abdomen—*not* your chest. When you exhale, pull your stomach muscles in. This is awkward in the beginning and the opposite from the way you normally breathe, but it *is* the technique for proper breathing, and with practice you will begin to feel comfortable with it. Okay, now put the book down and practice on your own for two or three minutes.

Do you feel a little light-headed from your new method of breathing? This is completely normal and shows that you're breathing properly. Nevertheless, many people have a tendency to breathe in too rapidly. Feeling slightly light-headed is fine, feeling dizzy is not. For most people, the simple act of slowing down the breathing process dispels any sensation of dizziness.

You should practice these breathing techniques several times throughout the day and again when you go to bed at night. At bedtime spend 5 to 15 minutes focusing only on deep breathing and nothing else. Don't worry about whether or not you will fall asleep—when practicing your deep breathing at night, try to stay awake. Practicing, not sleeping, will make you proficient at the technique. The more you use this technique, the more effective it will become as a tension reliever. Once you become comfortable with this method, you can use it anywhere. Try it the next time you get angry with a co-worker, get stuck in traffic or in a long line at the grocery store. Deep breathing is an excellent technique to use anytime you feel impatient or frustrated.

MUSCLE TENSION

Another often-ignored problem area for the insomniac is the muscles on either side of the neck that continue down into the top of the shoulders. In tense, nervous individuals, these muscles are usually tight and rigid. And since most insomniacs fall into this category as well, they too experience tense muscles. You can tell if this is a problem area for you by observing your body. Study your posture. Are your shoulders slightly elevated? Now relax your shoulders and see if they drop at least an inch. Now scan the rest of your body. Are your legs crossed, your arms folded, and are you clenching your teeth? Are you tapping one foot nervously? Are you frowning? Maybe not right now—although most of you will be later.

Begin doing body scans periodically throughout your day. Check your body with your mind's eye—are you holding it tight and rigid, as if some perceived threat lurks around the next corner? We want you to begin practicing letting go. Allow your shoulders to drop and uncross your legs. Stop gripping the steering wheel or hunching over a hurried dinner. In short, practice awareness and know that the same tension that prevents sleep at night accumulates in your posture throughout the day.

Exercises for Daily Practice

1. Deep breathing—three times daily a minimum of four consecutive breaths and 5 to 15 minutes upon retiring.
2. Body scan—two times daily practicing body awareness.
3. Body massage—Contrary to popular opinion, your body can respond to self-massage as efficiently as it would to an experienced masseuse.

   Focus on the muscles in your temple and jaw area, in your neck and shoulders, and in your upper arm. Use a small, circular motion, applying deep pressure as you go. Your muscles will love you for it.
4. Beginning with limited motion, gradually build up to the following exercise to prevent muscle strain to your neck. If you have suffered injury to this area, get medical clearance before proceeding. Without elevating your shoulders, bend your head to both sides, as if trying to touch your ear to your shoulders. Then bend your head forward and backward. While your head is backward, gently open and close your mouth. Do not rotate your head in this exercise as this can be irritating to the vertebrae in your neck, resulting in stiffness and discomfort.
5. Roll your shoulders forward with a very slow, exaggerated movement. As you do so, pull your head down toward your chest. Now reverse your shoulder movement by rolling your shoulders backward in a slow, circular motion, remembering to keep your head tilted forward.

The self-massage and shoulder exercises should be done at least twice a day, if not more, and particularly at bedtime. As you practice these exercises, your muscles will begin to let go of their chronic tension. Depending upon the individual, this gradual loosening-up process may take anywhere from two weeks to a month. Once achieved, however, your muscles will remain loose and flexible as long as you continue to do the above exercises. And remember, loose and supple muscles mean relaxation and a better night's sleep.

WHITE NOISE

We recommend that at least once a day you practice deep breathing to soft music or white noise. White noise is any pleasant and monotonous sound that blocks the bustle of the busy world. It can be the sound of a fan, a ticking clock, a tape of ocean sounds, or gentle rain. Allow yourself to feel the unchanging rhythm and to lose yourself in its monotony. It may be that you prefer it quiet when you practice, which is fine, since some people respond better to silence.

When you listen to your choice of sound, remember that bedtime is an excellent time to practice. Surprisingly, other family members not only enjoy, but benefit from, getting in on the act as well. Television, however, does not constitute white noise. We recommend, therefore, that you do not practice techniques with it on. Television is distracting and not at all conducive to a state of relaxation!

As you practice your breathing techniques to the sound of quiet music or white noise, focus only on your breathing. And imagine, if you will, that you are breathing in peace and relaxation, and breathing out the tension acquired throughout your busy day.

Selective Reverie—Session Number 2

Selective reverie is the process of using your imagination as an aid to relaxation. When done correctly, this type of visual imagery generates the production of alpha brain waves—a key element for deep relaxation. As you become proficient in this form of relaxation therapy, you will be able to stimulate greater alpha wave production. This, in turn, results in increasingly deeper states of relaxation.

When practiced daily, selective reverie enables you to develop an enriched mental capacity. Your mind becomes the canvas upon which you have total control over what you create. Selective reverie enhances physical and mental functioning by creating a positive working environment for all body systems. It is successfully used in the management of anxiety and phobias, and in pain control. Not only is it a successful technique for stress management, it is also an effective tool for controlling insomnia. Sports teams use this same process to enhance their playing power and great ideas get their start as creative imagery. Although you may question the power that lies in selective reverie, those who succeed do not. They use it as the foundation of achievement.

To begin practicing this technique as a sleep aid, you must allow your mind to engage in positive focus periodically throughout your day. Whether or not you believe it, begin visualizing yourself sleeping with ease. In your mind's eye, picture yourself asleep in your own bed—warm, comfortable, breathing rhythmically, peacefully. Allow this image to pass through your mind several times each day. Do not try to force yourself to believe this scene—just visualize it, as if you're looking down on yourself from above.

The second requirement in this process involves your nighttime exercise (although this can be done anytime you want to experience deep relaxation). When lying in bed spend several minutes deep breathing, then with eyes closed allow yourself to create a gentle scene on your mental canvas. To help you get started, we have created just such a scene for you. This is an example of the type of imagery you, too, can create.

> Imagine yourself lying in a feather bed with a soft warm comforter tucked under your chin. A fire crackles across the room and dancing shadows move dreamily about, caressing you with a warm golden glow. Outside, through frosted glass, you see the first snowfall of the year, gently enveloping, protecting all that lies beneath. And wafting up the stairs and through your open bedroom door strays the aroma of the fresh-baked cookies your grandma promised you. You feel yourself start to spin, gently drifting into sleep—warm and very, very secure.

An important step to successful guided imagery involves the use of four of your senses: sight, smell, hearing, and touch. Look at the example we just gave you. You can see how we incorporated sensory imagery into this mental script. This is the means by which selective reverie transcends the simple use of imagination. By including sight, touch, smell, and sound in your visualization, you are making it a total body experience. By incorporating these four senses into your imagery of peace and tranquillity, the antistress response of your body will be more profound.

What is the most beautiful, peaceful, and secure scene you can imagine? If you're floating in a boat on a small lake that you remember from your childhood, don't stop there. What kind of day is it? Is the sky deep blue or is it filled with coral clouds caressed by a setting sun? Has there just been a gentle rain, perhaps? Can you smell the fresh aroma of dampened earth? Or is a blanket of dusk covering your world with the sound of cicadas singing their evening song? You reach over the side of the boat and feel cool, silken water swirl lazily about your fingers. Remember, you must focus on nonstimulating imagery. Fantasizing that you have won the lottery is *not* conducive to sleep!

If your mind wanders, you may want to visualize a mental stop sign. Picture the sign in vivid detail. Make note of its bright red and white coloring. See its octagonal shape. And, in a loud mental voice, tell yourself, Stop. Then return to your creative fantasy. In time and with practice, the need to redirect becomes less and less. As your ability to concentrate improves, so will your ability to paint elaborate mental scripts.

You should also use the technique of resignation that we discussed in chapter 5. When oppositional thoughts occur, accept them. Don't get emotional by accusing yourself of not being capable of creative fantasy. Accept that these thoughts are there and then use your stop sign. Developing skill in this area is much like learning to master the technique of a piece of music. Although it will take time to play the piece proficiently, each time you practice, it sounds a little better than the time before.

Now it's your turn. Put the book down and give it a try. It's best if you practice in a comfortable chair or on your bed. First spend a minute or two deep breathing and then begin. Try for five minutes. If your mind wanders, use your stop sign.

How did you do? Did your mind rebel with numerous intrusive thoughts? Did you feel rather uptight as you tried to force yourself to be creative? Well, then you're on the right track! Rare is the person who initially has the mind control to take this kind of inward journey. It's like playing a musical instrument, or riding a bike for the first time. It takes practice to become proficient, to regain the lost creativity of childhood (it's more important that we learn how to give ourselves ulcers over a traffic jam!). With practice, however, not only will you get better at it, but you will begin to see results.

Do not become discouraged if you find that you are unable to concentrate on any type of fantasy imagery. An untrained mind has little patience and tries to resist concentration. It has been our experience that it takes an average of one to three weeks for a person to develop a sense of mastery over creative visualization. It appears, however, that once an adult learns to creatively fantasize, this remains a lifelong ability. People report that not only has selective reverie made them more adept at falling asleep, but it has also made them more creative on the job.

Selective reverie stimulates brain cells that may have been dormant since childhood. This type of mental stimulation not only enhances your level of creativity, but the very act of thinking itself. By activating dormant brain cells, you can increase overall brain function by boosting the percentage of brain matter that you use. As you gain new knowledge, you make connections between active and inactive brain cells. This, in turn, stimulates inactive cells into becoming functional brain cells. It is a process by which you can enhance healthy brain function well into old age. New and stimulating mental activities can promote vital brain capacity throughout your lifetime.

As you practice visualization be as creative as you like, however, never engage in any imagery that is negative in content. This is an uplifting exercise which promotes self-healing, not pessimistic thinking. If you worry about the aggravations of your day and have difficulty letting go of these nagging thoughts as you practice, you may find the following helpful. Before you begin to creatively fantasize, gather all of your concerns of the day and place them in the basket of a multicolored hot air balloon and allow it to set sail. Visualize your problems disappearing into the sky—disappearing for the 30 minutes you spend practicing your techniques. If you decide that you want to retrieve them at the end of your session, simply bring your balloon back to you. We guarantee that your troubles will be there waiting inside.

Symbolically, letting go of your problems before you begin your visualization can often free your mind for greater concentration and creativity.

Progressive Relaxation—Session Number 3

Progressive relaxation is an exercise in which you stretch, tense, and then release particular muscle groups throughout your body. This exercise requires muscle action as opposed to the passive release gained through autogenic relaxation addressed in Session Number 6. This is an easier exercise than autogenics and serves to prepare you for the methodology in your last biofeedback session.

To begin your initial practice session in progressive relaxation, assume a comfortable position, either lying down or sitting. It is best to have your arms at your side and your legs uncrossed. Take a slow, deep breath, breathing in relaxation and breathing out the accumulated tension of your day. Take two or three more deep breaths, breathing slowly and deeply at a rate that is comfortable for you.

Now, stretch the muscles in your right arm. When you feel the muscles pulling, make a tight fist and tense the muscles throughout your arm. Hold the tension to the slow count of five (adjust the count accordingly if this feels too tiring). Now, at the end of five, slowly release the tension in your fist and arm and let these muscles feel loose and limp. Notice the contrast between tense, tight muscles and the loose sensation in your relaxed arm. Now do the same procedure with your left arm.

Next take a deep breath and tighten the muscles in your back.

Hold to the count of five and then gently release your breath. As you completely empty your lungs, simultaneously allow the muscle tension to drain from your back and chest.

Now focus on your abdominal muscles. Tighten them to the count of five and then release.

Next move to your pelvic area and buttocks, and repeat the same tightening and releasing procedure.

Now move your focus down to your legs. While stretching both legs pull your toes down toward the floor. Tighten the muscles in your legs and hold to the slow count of five and then release. Allow the muscles to feel loose, limp, and relaxed.

Finally, you can focus on your neck and scalp. To attain the tension levels needed for this area, you can press your head into a pillow or the back of your chair. You will feel the tension in direct proportion to how hard you exert pressure. Maintain this pressure for the count of five and then relax. Next tighten the muscles in your facial area by scrunching your face and clenching your teeth. Once again hold to the count of five—and release, letting your teeth part as you do.

If at any point while stretching and tensing the muscles throughout your body you find that it becomes painful, *stop.* Just pass that group, take a slow, deep breath, and move on to the next muscle group.

Technique is not as important as feeling the contrast between a stretched, tight muscle and a limp, loose, and relaxed muscle. Spend four or five days practicing this particular exercise in order to get the feel of it, but realize its importance is merely preparatory for what is to follow.

Sensory Autogenics—Session Number 4

This session is the meat of this chapter. The following procedure is your replacement tool for the expensive electronic machinery used in biofeedback clinics. You will learn to use this monitoring mechanism to determine the level of your relaxation. The technique is simple, so simple in fact that people often think it is too easy to be effective. The ease of the technique is deceptive, however, because to gain mastery and benefit from it you must practice a minimum of four times weekly.

First, we want to explain the process of using body sensations as your monitoring source for determining depth of relaxation. Your body signals can provide the same feedback information as the electronic equipment available in professional settings. In some instances, your body may even provide greater accuracy as a measure of muscle relaxation. Although your body's sensations can be profound, you will adjust gradually to them. And not only will you adjust, but you will learn to enjoy them as you progress from one stage to the next. This approach offers an easy and smooth transition that promises to be fun, relaxing, and sleep inducing.

Table 4 shows you the various stages of relaxation and their associated sensation responses.

Table 4: Sensory Response

Stage of Relaxation	Associated Body Response	Level of Relaxation
Stage 1	Tingling hands and feet; heaviness in arms and legs; may have some difficulty concentrating. Continue to be aware of external stimuli.	Mild, slight therapeutic benefit.
Stage 2	Numbness to elbows and in feet; sensation of extreme heaviness throughout body; less aware of outside stimuli; facial muscles feel flaccid; breathing slow and regular.	Moderate, with tension release noted.
Stage 3	Increased numbness to include arms and legs; sensation of floating; possible muscle jerking; facial numbness may be present; complete internal psychological focus; sleep probable if effort not made to remain awake.	Deep, therapeutic relief achieved.
Stage 4	Total body numbness; some may become aware of heartbeat; pulse slows, blood pressure drops slightly; psychological focus narrowed (as in awareness of heartbeat); sense of peace and relaxation.	Deep, small endorphin release; mind and body healing; mild pain relief.
Stage 5	Total body numbness with floating feeling and sensation of turning in space; internal visualization occurs with a profound sense of relaxation; profound, large endorphin release; moderate pain relief.	Deep healing for mind and body.

Your goal is to be able to achieve Stage 4 and Stage 5 at will, independent of external factors. As you learn the technique of sensory autogenics, you will be able to gauge your level of relaxation based upon the body sensations you achieve. Most people can reach Stage 3 relaxation in about one month. The average individual can attain Stages 4 and 5 in two to three months. By the time a person reaches Stage 6, sleep is mastered and he or she has significantly reduced his or her stress level, as well. This is also an excellent management tool for pain control. It offers an effective alternative to a heavy pain medication regimen for those suffering from chronic pain.

Throughout the day your muscles are continually sending sensations of muscle tension and movement to your brain via sensory nerves. When, for instance, a muscle cramps or you have a headache, your brain interprets this as pain. Your brain can also interpret an overload of muscle tension as emotional tension. The interpretation of muscle senses can also be one of pleasure and relaxation—when, for example, you receive a massage or the pleasure perceived in your muscles while stretching.

As your muscles relax, however, the nerve endings cease to fire as rapidly and the signals from your muscles to your brain become weaker. As a result, you begin to develop the phenomena described in table 4. It is during Stage 5 that your muscle signals are the weakest of all. As a result, you cease to perceive body awareness or posturing. This is the reason that people in Stage 5 often report a turning-in-space sensation.

These body sensations are nothing mysterious. They are merely a result of muscles minus tension and represent a state of profound relaxation. Since few people ever feel this tension-free, most initially find these sensations strange and different.

The internal visualization that occurs in Stage 5 is a process similar to that achieved during profound muscle relaxation. Muscle relaxation and the production of alpha waves work in tandem to allow the firing rate of the brain cells to slow. Just as the reduced signals from your muscles produce a turning-in-space sensation, the slowed brain activity results in sensations of its own. Actually, however, it is the lack of sensation that the brain interprets as visualization. When you first enter Stage 5 the visual signals produced from relaxing neurons may produce subtle blue lines or a soft colored glow.

As relaxation deepens, the internal visualization unfolds, producing an array of colorful visions, almost dreamlike in quality. These visions lack the storyline of dreams, however, and resemble more the content of soft pastel paintings. Some people report seeing fields of colorful blooms or the cool, lush greenness of a garden setting.

It is during this stage of relaxation that endorphin production is at its highest. As a result, the healing impact upon one's mental and physical well-being is significant. If you can fall asleep during Stage 1 you have achieved your goal; however, striving for Stage 5 is a bonus well worth your effort.

You probably suffer from an overabundance of stress in your life. Consequently, your muscles are continually sending excess sensory signals to your brain. This tension may be long-standing and, as a result, your brain may no longer recognize it as muscle tension. Instead, you may interpret this excessive stimulation as generalized nervousness and anxiety.

As you begin the techniques that enable you to achieve the various stages of relaxation, keep the following in mind. Whether in Stage 1 or Stage 5, you are in total control. Should the telephone ring or someone knock at your door, you will be completely responsive. At any point there is muscle movement or a noise that you perceive as important, your body's nerve endings once again begin spending signals to your brain. This results in an alert and active mind.

Intense body sensations do not represent a loss of control. To the contrary, this is a learned skill that increases body awareness. It gives you mastery over a lifestyle that obstructs your ability to sleep, making you tense and uptight and preventing you from being as effective as you can be.

To begin autogenic exercises, you should assume the same comfortable position you used for progressive relaxation: arms at your side, legs uncrossed, comfortably sitting or lying down. If you like, spend a minute or two tensing and releasing the major muscle groups in your body. Then begin slow, deep breathing, three or four times—breathing in peace and relaxation and breathing out tension.

You follow the same systematic approach with autogenic exercises as you do with progressive relaxation. Unlike the physical activity of tensing muscle groups, however, autogenics involves the passive mental process of *imagining* these muscle groups feeling heavy and warm, and keeping very still as you do.

We recommend that you spend three or four days practicing the autogenic technique in the following manner. Repeat the phrase: "My (body part) feels heavy and warm" three times (more if necessary) and very slowly. Move throughout your body using a systematic approach, focusing on each area for at least 30 seconds. Progress lazily from the tip of your toes to the very top of your head.

As you become increasingly proficient, your approach can vary. Some people begin with their lower body, imagining a warm wave of relaxation engulfing their feet, then washing gently up around their calves—warm, swirling water, relaxing, soothing. Some prefer using imagery such as a warm blanket of relaxation being pulled up slowly over their body, covering first their feet, then moving slowly up over their legs—warm, soft, filling each body part it covers with peace, heaviness, relaxation, and warmth. You may prefer beginning with your hands, moving slowly up your arms to your shoulders, into your chest muscles, abdomen, back muscles, and down into the legs and feet. Lastly, always remember facial, neck, and scalp areas. Whatever approach is effective for you is the one you should use.

For the sake of instruction, however, begin with your feet and slowly progress upward through your body. Remember that the common denominator for this type of exercise is the terminology. It is important to concentrate on two words throughout your practice sessions: heavy and warm.

After you feel comfortable with the basic technique of imagining body parts as feeling heavy and warm, you can become creative and begin using your selective reverie techniques. For example, you may imagine yourself lying on a warm, golden beach on a private tropical island, where you can imagine the warmth of the sun penetrating your muscles. You hear the sound of pounding surf, you can almost taste the warm salt air, you visualize a lone sea gull soaring overhead.

Begin this imagery immediately after your initial deep breathing. And remember, as you create your imagery, include your senses of touch, smell, taste (if appropriate), and hearing. Spend about five minutes focusing on this scene and then begin your autogenic exercises. Continue to imagine yourself on the beach, for example, but narrow your sensory focus to the perception of warmth from the sun, feeling it penetrating each muscle group and making that particular part feel heavy and warm.

As you imagine the warmth of the sun penetrating your muscles, repeat slowly within your mind:

> My feet feel warmth from the sun, and the warmth is making my feet feel heavy. My feet are heavy and warm. I feel the heat from the sun penetrating deeply into my feet—warm and soothing. My feet feel heavy and heavier and now I feel this warmth

spreading upward into the muscles of my calves. I feel warmth—
and the muscles are feeling heavy and heavier.

Progress this way upward throughout your entire body, visualizing the warmth of the sun soothing and relaxing your muscles as you go. Remember, you should spend at least 30 seconds on each body section, progressing in pairs as you do. Focus on both feet, for example, then your calves, up into both thighs, then into your buttocks and pelvic area. Then concentrate on the abdominal and chest muscles, moving next into your back and spinal area. Progress upward into your shoulders, and then focus on your arms. And remember not to forget your hands. Lastly, feel the penetrating warmth in your neck, your scalp, and then all the little muscles in your face.

If you have difficulty imagining warmth, think back to a time when you were lying in the sun, or were relaxing in a boat fishing, mesmerized by the dragonfly as it danced on the tip of your pole. Think back—visualize—you can almost feel the heat of the sun as you remember this scene. Don't try to force your muscles to feel heavy and warm, however. If you find that your mind resists these suggestions, just try to imagine how heavy and warm muscles would feel. What would you feel right now if you were lying in the sun in a tropical paradise?

Use your imagination. If the beach isn't for you, imagine a warm, rustic cabin where you're relaxing in front of a dancing fire. Perhaps you prefer to float in a pool of warm, swirling water. Whatever scenes produce the greatest sense of warmth for you should be your focus.

You can easily master this technique with consistent practice. As you gain skill, you'll find that you quickly enter the deepest stages of relaxation with very little effort on your part (you may need only 10 seconds per muscle group).

When you master autogenics and use the technique along with the active management techniques outlined in chapters 4 and 5, you will have gained the skills to promote positive mental health and sound restful sleep.

Body Temperature—Session Number 5

When you feel agitated or nervous, certain physiological responses occur. Your muscles become tight, your heart and respiratory rates increase, and there is an activation of all organ systems. As a result, blood flow is shunted from your skin and directed toward your deep, large muscles and vital organs. This prepares you for the natural fight or flight response that begins to address the stimuli that are causing stress in your life. Whether you are being pursued by a dark shadow in the night, are having an argument with your mother-in-law, or have just lost your paycheck, your body will respond in the manner described above. Your brain interprets stress as a need for a fight or flight response. Most of life's stressors, however, are more subtle. It may be stress encountered from a two-hour stint in rush hour traffic, an insensitive remark from a co-worker, or the simple realization that the laugh lines around your mouth are anything but funny. Unfortunately, accumulation of such stressors by day's end are hardly conducive to deep and restful sleep.

Since blood has an average temperature of 99.6 degrees Fahrenheit, it helps keep you warm as it circulates through the capillaries in your skin. When you feel nervous, tense, or angry, however, the blood leaves your skin and heads for your body's organs and large muscles. When this occurs, people typically experience a sensation of chilliness (see table 5).

Table 5: Skin Temperature

Below 80 degrees	80 to 84 degrees	85 to 89 degrees
Extreme tension	Moderate tension	Mild tension

90 to 94 degrees	Over 95 degrees
Moderate relaxation	Deep relaxation

When individuals take steroids, tranquilizers, hypertensive medications, alcohol, or any form of nicotine, skin temperature may not reflect accurate tension levels.

In a clinical setting, a therapist determines your tension level by attaching a thermal sensor to your index finger at the beginning of the biofeedback session. Ideally, at the conclusion of the session your finger temperature will have increased. As you relax, excess blood leaves muscles and organs and returns to the capillaries within your skin, indicating decreased tension levels. Although it is difficult to determine such exact finger temperature at home, you can employ a reasonable facsimile. A good standard by which you can measure finger temperature is to place your fingers on the front of your neck to the right or left of your Adam's apple. This particular spot maintains a consistent body temperature between 90 and 94 degrees Fahrenheit. If you'll refer to the chart, you'll notice this is the hand temperature range indicating a moderate level of relaxation.

Now touch this area of your neck. Do your fingers feel cool? You may be feeling mild tension. Are your fingers absolutely cold? Chances are you are feeling extremely tense. Or maybe your fingers feel warm against your neck. Unless the room is extremely warm, you are most likely feeling comfortable and relaxed.

Monitor your finger temperature before and after each practice session. Often, people are surprised to find when they begin learning these techniques their fingers are frequently cool. They may be having difficulty sleeping at night, but they are not aware that they are experiencing excess tension. If your fingers feel cool, do a body scan. You may find that you are feeling anxious after all. Your stomach feels tight, you're clenching your teeth, the muscles in your forehead feel tight, you're holding your shoulders high—all areas that you need to scan when your fingers feel cool.

The ability to increase finger temperature takes time to develop. Frequently, beginners complain of increased finger coolness after the first one to two weeks of autogenic practice. This happens to about 65 percent of those new to autogenics, so do not interpret this as a negative reaction should it occur. In actuality, this is a positive indicator of a person's ability to influence body temperature, an underdeveloped ability that with training gains positive control.

You cannot force your extremities to increase their temperature. This is a passive response. As you practice, just continue to focus on warming phrases and warm imagery. Try to imagine what warm hands feel like; what it feels like, for example, to hold cold hands in front of a camp fire. Or what about that cold rain that soaked you to the bone? You came home, climbed into a steaming hot shower and never felt such marvelous, penetrating warmth in your life! What did that feel like? Let your mind trick your body into warming itself. You can't force it to respond, however, because your body will rebel and attempt to do the opposite. Simply enjoy your fantasy of warmth and do not worry whether or not you are doing the job correctly.

If you continue with patient practice, you will develop the ability to alter your body's negative response to stress. The approaches to stress and insomnia management outlined in this book are more than just tools: They provide a means for lifestyle changes that enable you to direct your energy toward wellness. If you apply these techniques consistently, you can gain healthful mastery over what you previously thought you had little control.

Troubleshooting—Session Number 6

This last session discusses a few obstacles you may encounter during your biofeedback and guided imagery sessions.

TENSION

Many people complain of added tension when they begin practicing relaxation techniques. Some continue to have difficulty falling asleep or complain of headaches. Others notice increased tightness in the head and shoulder muscles. These are all examples of trying too hard.

Remember, you're not supposed to put pressure on yourself to force relaxation, as this is a gentle letting go process. This is a time to be kind to you. We become so accustomed to life demanding from us that somehow we feel our world isn't functioning properly if it isn't filled with tension and pressure. It is worth 30 minutes a day, however, to try to change your approach to dealing with this kind of tension, tension that not only prevents you from sleeping at night, but prevents you from enjoying life in general.

When you practice these techniques, put a hold on demand. For 30 minutes you are going to let go. Make a promise to yourself that you will not worry about getting to sleep, feeling relaxed, or whether or not you feel warm. For 30 minutes none of that really matters. Ship all of your concerns and cares of the day on your hot air balloon, and give yourself 30 minutes of freedom.

So, if you feel increased tension, it's okay. If you worry about it, it will last longer than if you don't. Either way, your tension will gradually diminish. For the average person, however, tension levels often begin to decrease within the second week.

CONCENTRATION

Some people report that they cannot concentrate on their exercises. They try, but find that their mind continually wanders. Again, stop worrying, this is okay. Without berating yourself, gently try to pull your mind back to target. In time you will find that this simple act of directing your mind becomes easier. It becomes easier not only regarding relaxation training, but in other tasks as well. You are training your mind in much the same manner as a weight trainer develops his or her muscles. Results take time to show! If, however, poor concentration is a problem for you in other areas of your life, it may be wise for you to speak to your family physician. Concentration difficulties can be a result of depression, which a mental health professional can often treat easily and effectively.

BACKTRACKING

It's a common and normal concern to believe you are backtracking. You might be making progress when suddenly, not only does progress appear to stop, but you feel like you're regressing. Often, this means you have reached a level of greater self-understanding. As a result, you experience a heightened awareness of new and subtle stress responses to your relaxation training.

As you reach plateaus or have periods of poor progress, *stop*. Scan your body and your emotional state. You may find that it's time to incorporate a newly surfaced stress response into your training program. Challenge your reaction to this new stressor in your thought journal. Retake the mood awareness profile (see page 28) to determine the impact it is having on your emotional state. Deal with each new stressor that surfaces as you dealt with the first. As time passes, it becomes increasingly easy to work through these new problems as they arise. As your tension level decreases, you will problem solve more effectively. In addition, you will become more efficient at letting go of the stress that accompanies these problems.

THE TRYING ERROR

Some people report that they still have trouble trying to fall asleep, even with relaxation exercises. Keep in mind that as long as you *try* to fall asleep you are not doing anything different from what you have done in the past. It didn't work then and it won't work now. When you climb into bed at night to do your 30 minutes of exercises, *do not* try to fall asleep. During your practice session you are to remain awake. The purpose of relaxation training is to learn how to let go of stress—and you can't learn if you're asleep. Only as you develop your ability to release stress and tension will your autonomic nervous system become free from intrusions and pave the way for natural sleep to occur.

HYPNIC JERKS

Hypnic jerks are another frequent complaint. We've all experienced this normal limb-jerking or body-jumping sensation before falling asleep or during a period of deep relaxation. They merely indicate disengagement of the nervous system from an alert state to a relaxed or sleep state, and are nothing you should fear. During this period, voluntary muscle control is suddenly and rapidly lost, resulting in muscle jerks.

ALPHA WAVES

Throughout your practice session, keep your eyes gently closed. By simply opening your eyes during relaxation training you can stimulate the production of beta waves. These rapid brain waves can interrupt the cycle of relaxation, producing an alert and active mind. The mere act of closing your eyes, however, is sufficient to begin producing alpha waves—the pattern associated with tranquillity and quietness. Closing your eyes may not be enough to reduce all of your stress and tension, but it can enhance the effectiveness of other relaxation techniques. Remember, when you open your eyes even briefly during your practice sessions, you interrupt the production of relaxing alpha waves.

REACTIVATION

Some people report feeling groggy after their practice sessions. You can avoid this, however, if you reactivate. Begin by stretching your arms and legs and then slowly open your eyes. Sit or lie quietly for another 30 seconds, stand, then stretch again. You can then resume normal activity, refreshed and relaxed. When some people do not reactivate, they have a tendency to feel groggy for 10 or 15 minutes afterward.

Chapter 7
Nature's Remedies as Sleep Aids

As health care costs continue to climb and people become increasingly aware of the need to prevent disease instead of just treat it, many are beginning to take responsibility for their health and focus on wellness. Changing attitudes reflect a heightened awareness of the role of prevention and a search for non-invasive measures that can improve the overall quality of life. In addition to biofeedback, the following natural measures are excellent and gentle tools effective not only for healthy sleep management, but for peoples' overall mental and physical health as well.

VALERIAN

Known as valerian or garden heliotrope, this herb shows no ill effects and is safe for use as a mild tranquilizer. It is currently approved as a food additive and is available in most health food stores in capsule and teabag form. The tranquilizing effects of this herb are due to its active ingredient, valepotriates.

Unfortunately, there is not a standard amount of the herb which is known to be effective, since the strength of the active ingredient varies from one plant to the next. Trial and error becomes your best means of determining the amount that is right for you.

It is recommended, however, that you limit your daily intake to two cups of valerian tea at bedtime. If you decide to use capsules, take a maximum of 900 milligrams 30 minutes before retiring.

CARBOHYDRATES

If you want to quiet shaky nerves that can prevent you from sleeping at night, you can snack on carbohydrates before going to bed. A nighttime snack of rice cakes, plain white bread, or a few saltines can do much to promote sleep. Few people realize the negative impact that a heavy evening meal rich in protein and fat can have on the body's ability to achieve restful sleep.

When you eat carbohydrates, your pancreas quickly releases insulin, which not only controls blood sugar levels but performs other functions, as well. One of these is its ability to decrease the concentration of amino acids circulating within the bloodstream. The only amino acid that insulin appears to have no effect upon is L-Tryptophan, the amino acid which the brain uses to manufacture serotonin. Serotonin helps reduce feelings of tension and stress and aids in the promotion of sleep. Since carbohydrates cause the pancreas to decrease other amino acid levels within the bloodstream, L-Tryptophan does not have to compete with these amino acids to gain entry into the brain. Therefore, greater amounts of L-Tryptophan can enter the brain.

It is important that only carbohydrates be eaten, however. The proverbial glass of milk won't do because the fat and protein content of milk interfere with L-Tryptophan's ability to reach the brain. If protein is eaten in conjunction with a carbohydrate snack, insulin will not be as effective. As a result, other amino acids will enter the brain and reduce the amount of L-Tryptophan that can enter. Fats, on the other hand, slow down the whole process of digestion, thus significantly delaying the entry of L-Tryptophan into the brain.

You should become aware of the tranquilizing effects of carbohydrates within 30 minutes of eating your bedtime snack. We recommend, however, that you wait at least three hours after a heavy meal to eat this snack to prevent interference from the fats and proteins in your last meal.

You should not confuse the L-Tryptophan present in the foods you eat with that which can be purchased in tablet form. it is the tablet form of this amino acid that the FDA has banned for public consumption. The deaths that have occurred from the use of L-Tryptophan tablets and capsules should not be associated with naturally occurring L-Tryptophan found in a healthy diet.

Finally, several other factors can contribute to insomnia. Many people take vitamins to enhance their sense of vitality, and to replace what they feel may be missing in their diets. What most people don't realize, however, is vitamin E, often in doses as low as 200 I.U., may contribute to insomnia. For reasons that remain unclear, vitamin E can cause restlessness in susceptible individuals. If you suspect that this may be a problem for you, stop taking vitamin E. Within three days it will be out of your system and for some people this means a better night's sleep. You can then experiment and reduce the dosage to a level that does not interrupt your sleep.

It's an absolute necessity to abstain from caffeine if you want to treat your insomnia effectively. This includes hidden caffeine such as that found in chocolate, soda, certain brands of pain relievers and even decaffeinated coffee. You must begin reading labels and adjust your diet accordingly. For the insomniac, caffeine is poison, and you must avoid even the minuscule amounts that are found in decaffeinated coffee!

AEROBIC CONDITIONING

Exercise remains one of the reasons that insomnia runs rampant in technological societies. Although the requirements of modern living demand a great deal of mental energy, the need for hard physical labor is gone. This may represent progress, but it exacts a price. Most people have excess stress in their lives as a result of the mental demands placed upon them. Frequently, however, they turn to negative stress relievers such as alcohol, food, drugs, or temper tantrums to manage this stress. It is little wonder that accumulated stress combined with poor problem-solving skills produces insomnia.

You may be thinking that this is true enough, but on top of all your psychological stress you don't stop moving, either. Does your constant motion, however, ever produce 20 or 30 minutes of nonstop huffing and puffing? Chances are, it does not. This leads us into a discussion about aerobic conditioning—a panacea for your stress overload and sleepless nights.

Aerobic conditioning results when you maintain an accelerated and sustained heart and respiration rate for 20 to 30 minutes, a minimum of four times weekly. The physical demands placed on your muscles and the added oxygen intake serve as an excellent stress reducer and sleep enhancer. It is more than this, however, as aerobic activity stimulates the production and release of the brain chemical endorphin. In conjunction with muscle exertion, endorphin release promotes an increased sense of calm and well-being, and a greater ability to tolerate stress. The benefits from aerobic conditioning extend throughout your day and into the night by encouraging deep, restful sleep with a general reduction in falling asleep time.

The benefits from aerobic fitness are many. If you're still not convinced that a brisk walk, jumping rope, or aerobic dancing are for you, read over the following list. Aerobic conditioning can result in:

1. Reduced resting heartbeat with ability to pump blood more efficiently
2. An increase in the number, size, and elasticity of blood vessels promoting better circulation
3. A lowered cholesterol and triglyceride (fats) level within the blood
4. A decrease in blood clot formation thus lowering the risk for stroke and heart attack
5. Weight loss and lowering of blood pressure
6. The ability of the body to use oxygen more efficiently
7. Lower blood sugar levels resulting in less blood sugar being converted to triglycerides
8. A decrease in stress hormone (adrenaline) production
9. An increased tolerance of stress
10. A reduction in symptoms of depression with improved concentration
11. Deeper, more restful sleep

If you are interested in beginning an aerobic exercise program, it is important that you adhere to the guidelines in the following chart:

Age	Sustained Target Heart Rate Range
20	135 to 165
30	130 to 160
35	127 to 153
40	124 to 150
45	120 to 145
50	115 to 140
55	110 to 135
60	105 to 130
65	100 to 128
70	95 to 120

We recommend that anyone over 35 years of age or with an existing medical condition receive clearance from his or her physician before engaging in an exercise program.

SLEEP DEPRIVATION THERAPY

Another approach to treating depression involves the use of sleep deprivation; however, you should have a medical examination and receive a clear bill of health before you try this method. Most depressed people suffer no ill effects from this therapy, and many experience a general improvement in mood. This method should not replace professional mental health consultation.

The technique is not complicated. Simply stay awake all night! We do not recommend that you try this during your work week or when you may have to operate machinery (including driving your car). However, you can use sleep deprivation to fight your depression on a weekend or during other free time.

Do not be afraid that 24 hours without sleep will take you three days to recoup. It only takes one good night's sleep after staying up all night to awaken feeling rested (and less depressed). Even insomniacs manage an adequate night's sleep if completely sleep deprived for 24 hours. If, however, your depression becomes worse or you develop self-destructive tendencies, you should seek prompt mental health consultation.

Sleep deprivation may produce positive effects by increasing endorphin production, the body's natural painkiller and antidepressant. It appears that depressed individuals may have an abnormally low level of circulating endorphin. Sleep deprivation may stimulate an increase, resulting in a more positive and uplifted mood.

Chapter 8
The Older Adult and Insomnia

Approximately 85 percent of individuals ages 55 to 90 experience episodic insomnia. Although quality sleep does diminish somewhat as we age, insomnia is not an inevitable part of growing older. All of the techniques in this book apply to the older adult, but there are additional factors that apply as well. Although modern medicine offers numerous lifesaving techniques, an individual must assume the bulk of responsibility for promoting his own health. And, the best place for a person to begin to make this commitment to health is with his own attitude. Although uninterrupted sleep may be more difficult to achieve, insomnia may not be as much a factor in growing older as it is a by-product of a negative attitude about aging. The following is a list of special factors that contribute to the development of insomnia in older adults; but with a positive attitude and a commitment to improve one's overall health, you *can* overcome many of the obstacles that prevent quality sleep.

- Pain/medical disorders
- Restricted activity/decreased exercise
- Depression
- Increased daytime napping
- Medication reactions
- Age-associated decrease in ability to maintain sleep
- Age-associated reduction in depth of sleep
- Increased sleep-related breathing disorders
- The normal two- to-four-second mini-arousals that occur with young adults during sleep become much more pronounced and frequent with older adults. Although they may

not remember waking up, they can effect alertness and energy the following day.

Although the ability to sleep naturally diminishes with age, the need for sleep does not. It becomes paramount, therefore, that the older adult maintains a strict sleep/wake rhythm. The older adult should avoid daytime napping and maintain a bedtime regimen in which he or she goes to bed only when sleepy, but gets up at the same time each morning. The bedroom should be used only for sleep so that the troubled sleeper develops a strong association between bed and sleep. To further enhance the ability to achieve quality sleep, he or she should resist the urge to go to bed too early. In addition, the older adult should limit time in bed to a maximum of seven hours nightly.

Staying in bed for periods longer than seven hours increases the likelihood of prolonged wakefulness when the person goes to bed that same night. If, however, excessive daytime sleepiness becomes a problem, a brief 30-minute nap at the same time each day is often the perfect remedy.

Although all the techniques addressed throughout this book are beneficial for the older adult, an area of additional concern is the use of sleeping medications. Older adults comprise about 12 percent of the U.S. population, and yet they consume nearly 35 percent of the prescription drugs sold in any given year. Although sleeping pills are appropriate in some short-term situations, the older adult should not use them for extended periods, as the multiple risk factors associated with long-term use are even more pronounced for this age group.

Because of the naturally slowing metabolism that occurs with increasing age, the body does not handle medications as efficiently and, therefore, does not break them down or eliminate them as quickly. As a result, medication can accumulate in the body with potentially lethal results. This can produce symptoms of overdose due to the buildup of medications within the body. Adverse drug interactions can occur in addition to daytime sedation. Even symptoms of senility can develop in older adults if medications are not broken down or eliminated as quickly as they should. Some cases of age-related amnesia may be drug related as well. When properly withdrawn from psychotropic medications, some older adults may experience increased alertness and notice a marked improvement in memory.

We do not recommend benzodiazepines and hypnotics for

long-term use. For the older adult who remains unable to maintain sleep without medication, a low dose of one of the antidepressants can be helpful. Antidepressants cause less motor impairment, daytime sleepiness, and confusion than minor tranquilizers and hypnotic drugs. In addition, they do not produce drug tolerance. Antidepressants are beneficial for the large segment of the older population who suffer from depression as well as insomnia. However, physicians will not prescribe antidepressants unless they observe clearly demonstrated symptoms of depression. In addition, tricyclic antidepressants may also help the older adult who suffers from sleep apnea by diminishing his or her apneic episodes (see chapter 10). Tranquilizers, on the other hand, can increase the intensity of a nonbreathing episode. Antidepressants can initially produce some daytime sleepiness, however, this is usually short term, rarely lasting longer than one week.

Finally, sleep disturbances (and depression) are often a product of unstimulating and sedentary lifestyles. Aging is inevitable, but aging does not have to be synonymous with decay. The mind can stay young and have a positive influence on longevity and promote a more productive and independent lifestyle. Too often older adults focus on what was: when they were younger, when their children were small, and on those no longer living. This focus on yesterday robs an individual of his or her ability to live today. Likewise, it lends itself to depression, poor health, and an inability to maintain restful and healing sleep.

Some older adults need to challenge the negative image they have of themselves. The picture they carry in their minds is what they become. One of the first commitments an older adult can make is to get active—both physically and mentally—stimulating the mind with activities that focus on today. The older adult should be open to opportunities to become active within his or her range of capabilities.

Probably of even greater importance, however, is the need for physical activity. Although medical complications can reduce the overall physical capacity of a person, rarely do they prevent any or all movement. For the older adult, we recommend any type of physician-approved activity that causes the muscles to stretch, heart rate to increase above 100 beats per minute, and breathing to become more rapid. This aerobic activity will not only lessen depression, but will produce deeper and more restful sleep as well (see chapter 7). If one is to experience these benefits, however, one must make a commitment. Exercise sessions must last at least 20 minutes to keep the heart beating at a sustained rapid rate. In addition, one must exercise a minimum of three to four times weekly. Whether the exercise consists of a brisk walk, using a stationary cycle, or joining an older adults aerobic class, the result will be the same. After several weeks of consistent effort, the individual will experience a gradual improvement in mood, and sleep will become deeper with fewer nighttime awakenings.

With the increased sense of well-being that is a product of restful sleep, many people find that a zest for life replaces their focus on yesterday. A positive outlook not only improves the quality of today, but allows you to look forward to tomorrow.

Chapter 9
How Premenstrual Syndrome Affects Your Sleep Regimen

If you are a female of childbearing age you are likely bothered by cyclical changes in your body and mood that correlate closely with your menstrual cycles. Symptoms of premenstrual syndrome (PMS) begin shortly after ovulation, gradually increase, and reach their peak in intensity five or so days before menstruation begins. Once the menstrual period starts, symptoms soon diminish and one begins experiencing an increased sense of physical and mental well-being—usually by the second day of one's period. Although nearly 80 percent of all women experience some symptoms of PMS, less than 30 percent of these women experience symptoms severe enough to require medical attention. When a woman seeks professional help, however, it is the symptom-free period between the onset of menstruation and ovulation which aids the physician in making the diagnoses of PMS.

PMS increases with age, with peak severity occurring between ages 30 and 40 and subsiding after menopause. Women who have had hysterectomies, but have one or both ovaries remaining, can experience all of the symptoms of PMS as well.

SYMPTOMS

The list of symptoms is long and a woman may experience any combination of these symptoms. The following chart outlines what is only too familiar to many women:

Physical Symptoms	**Psychological Symptoms**
Abdominal bloating	Mood swings
Headaches	Aggression/Anger
Abdominal cramps	Depression
Leg aches	Irritability
Water retention	Forgetfulness
Painful breasts	Confusion
Constipation	Crying spells
Gastrointestinal upsets	Restlessness
Insomnia	
Fatigue	

CAUSES OF PMS

Although researchers have yet to determine a specific cause for PMS, they have identified several factors that appear to contribute to the problem. Research suggests that an excess of estrogen or a deficiency in progesterone may induce premenstrual symptoms. Also theorized as causal in producing the discomfort associated with PMS is fluid retention, hypoglycemia, and vitamin deficiencies. Stress, too, can induce symptoms of PMS: a miscarriage, childbirth, illness or surgery, the discontinuation of birth control pills, a divorce, the loss of a job or a loved one—whatever the individual, or her body, perceives as stressful may be sufficient to induce PMS.

At this point, however, research results remain inconclusive. It may be that stress in the physiologically predisposed woman is sufficient to produce PMS. Although it is impossible to eliminate all stress from these women's lives, they can build their line of defenses with proper nutrition, vitamin supplementation, and exercise. By maintaining optimum physical health, women suffering from PMS can lessen the severity of the symptoms that often increase with stress.

If you suffer from PMS, we have devoted the rest of this section to measures which will improve your physical health. The entire contents of this book, however, are as important for the PMS sufferer as for the insomniac. This book can help you deal more effectively with daily stress and the added emotional burden that PMS places on your life.

TREATMENT APPROACHES

Although premenstrual symptoms may never entirely subside, they can become manageable with a holistic treatment approach. If symptoms are severe, medical intervention may be necessary to include such prescribed medications as diuretics, antidepressants, or hormones such as progesterone and antiprostaglandins. If your condition requires medical supervision, you should use the principles outlined in this chapter in conjunction with your doctor's treatment. If symptoms are not of sufficient intensity to warrant medical attention, however, the following measures may prove adequate to lessen the pain and discomfort associated with PMS.

Vitamin Therapy
Many people are skeptical about the benefits of taking vitamins. Vitamin therapy is, after all, rarely the treatment of choice for most medical conditions. For PMS sufferers, however, vitamins appear to be one of the key elements, along with diet and exercise, for long term relief of discomfort. Unfortunately, the majority of people, including PMS sufferers, do not follow a consistent vitamin regimen. Yet many of these same people dismiss the possibility that vitamins can have a positive impact upon overall health—and PMS specifically.

You have nothing to lose if you follow the methods outlined in this chapter. You are already suffering from a monthly agony that can only improve if you apply a holistic approach to your health needs.

Pyridoxine
Pyridoxine or vitamin B6 helps regulate body fluids, thus reducing the bloating and water retention associated with PMS. Vitamin B6 aids in maintaining a balance between sodium and potassium within the body tissues. By supplementing your diet with 60 to 100 milligrams of vitamin B6 daily, you can reduce the fluid retention that causes weight gain, breast tenderness, and abdominal bloating.

Do not, however, think that because a little may be good, a lot will be better. Research indicates that doses larger than 400 milligrams daily may cause nerve damage. In addition, if you take some B vitamins by themselves (and B6 is one of them), they can produce symptoms of deficiency in the other B vitamins. Therefore, if you do add vitamin B6 to your diet, you should take a supplement that provides the entire B complex.

Many of the symptoms of a vitamin B deficiency are the same symptoms associated with PMS, producing fatigue, irritability, depression, nervousness, constipation, and insomnia. This is an extremely common deficiency in American society, since, overall, Americans eat too many processed foods lacking in B vitamins. Processed foods labeled enriched also lack many of the essential B vitamins and should be avoided. The PMS sufferer should also avoid sugar, caffeine, and alcohol as these, too, destroy the vitamin B content in food.

The vitamin B complex increases energy levels, protects the nervous system, and is an excellent stress supplement for anyone with a hectic lifestyle. In addition to supplementation, foods particularly rich in the B complex include wheat germ, blackstrap molasses, liver, and Brewer's yeast.

Niacin

Niacin, also a member of the B family, can be helpful for sleep, irritability, depression, and headaches—particularly migraine headaches. By taking 100 to 150 milligrams daily, you may begin to see some improvement in the above symptoms.

A unique reaction of niacin is its ability to stimulate peripheral circulation; however, this produces a side effect that can be somewhat frightening to the niacin newcomer. Approximately 15 minutes after taking this particular vitamin, most people experience an intense itching, tingling sensation and their bodies often turn beat red! Itching may affect various parts or all of the body and merely indicates stimulation of the body's peripheral circulation.

This sensation is proof that niacin is doing its intended job and is in no way harmful or dangerous. To the contrary, it is this very flushing that can reduce the pain of migraine headaches and improve a person's complexion. It normally subsides in 15 to 20 minutes.

If, however, this sensation is uncomfortable for you, you can take one of the synthetic forms of niacin that does not produce flushing: niacinamide or nicotinamide. Although they, too, help reduce irritability and improve sleep, they do not diminish the pain of a migraine headache. It is the flushing property of niacin that reduces the discomfort of migraines, and not the vitamin itself.

Choline

Choline, also a member of the B family, has been helpful in relieving insomnia and constipation. To achieve these effects, however, most people have had to take a dosage greater than the recommended daily allowance. Most people report that 500 milligrams to 1,000 milligrams daily is adequate to do the job.

Calcium

Everyone knows that calcium helps build strong bones and teeth, but it has other benefits as well, particularly for the PMS sufferer. Calcium is an excellent mineral to help calm nerves and promote sound, restful sleep. The body also needs it to help blood clot normally, so this can be a real plus for those plagued by extremely heavy periods. To achieve the benefits both for sleep and normal blood clotting, we recommend 1,200 milligrams nightly half an hour before bedtime.

Calcium supplements are available in two forms: calcium lactate and calcium gluconate. Since calcium lactate is assimilated more easily by the body, we recommend using this form of calcium.

Vitamin D

A vitamin D deficiency can result in insomnia, irritability, and an increased sensitivity to pain. In addition, you may experience muscle spasms, cramps, and increased bleeding. Vitamin D is also necessary to promote the assimilation of calcium. A deficiency in this particular vitamin can intensify the symptoms of PMS, so it is very important that adequate amounts of this vitamin are present within the body.

Vitamin D is unique in that the body manufactures it through an interaction of ultraviolet sunlight and ergosterol, an oily substance present on the skin. Through a complicated process, sunlight transforms ergosterol into vitamin D, which is then transferred through the skin and into the bloodstream. Unfortunately, long winters, smog, heavy clothing, and sedentary lifestyles which keep us indoors much of the time prevent the ability of our skin to come into contact with the sunlight necessary for vitamin D synthesis. Although almost everyone is aware of the hazards of too much sun, moderate exposure to sunshine is necessary. If this is not possible for you, taking 400 IU of vitamin D daily will meet minimum nutritional requirements.

Although some PMS sufferers have benefited from large doses up to 5,000 IU daily, vitamin D is a fat-soluble vitamin and accumulates in the body. If you take excessively large doses over a prolonged period, you may develop toxic levels of this vitamin that can be life threatening. We suggest, therefore, that you do not exceed 1,000 IU daily.

Vitamin K

Vitamin K promotes normal blood clotting, thus it can reduce excessive clotting or the flow in heavy or prolonged periods. It also appears that in some individuals vitamin K relieves pain, thereby reducing the discomfort associated with cramping.

Vitamin K is present in large amounts in spinach, cabbage, cauliflower, and other green leafy vegetables. Unfortunately, aspirin destroys vitamin K, which is the drug used most frequently by PMS sufferers. For women who are the unfortunate victims of PMS, 20 milligrams of vitamin K daily is usually enough to ease their discomfort.

Vitamin K is also a fat-soluble vitamin, so it should be taken cautiously. We recommend, therefore, that you increase your intake of foods rich in vitamin K in lieu of vitamin K tablets. A daily serving of one of the aforementioned vegetables usually provides your minimum daily requirements of this particular nutrient.

Diet and Exercise

PMS sufferers should avoid diets consisting of heavy protein and fatty foods. Instead, a healthy daily nutritional intake should contain at least 60 percent complex carbohydrates. Protein sources should consist primarily of poultry and fish with an overall diet high in fruits, vegetables, whole grains, and legumes. If you have difficulty abstaining permanently from alcohol, sugar, and caffeine, at least do so the week prior to the onset of menstruation.

Finally, beginning a daily, brisk walk program of 20 to 30 minutes duration can significantly reduce symptoms of PMS, including depression, insomnia, irritability, and menstrual cramping. Consistent exercise is of paramount importance for the effective management of PMS.

Chapter 10
Sleep Apnea

Sleep influences the regulation of nearly all of our physical and psychological functioning. Ideally, it recharges our batteries, restores healthy function and protects us from excessive wear and tear.

Unfortunately, for victims of sleep apnea, sleep is not a time of restoration, but a time of psychological and physical deterioration. This condition, characterized by episodes of non-breathing (apnea) or severely impaired breathing (hypoventilation), occurs during sleep. One of the key symptoms of this disorder, and one that should send up a red flag, is heavy, thunderous snoring. If you have five or more of the following symptoms and snore heavily, you, too, may be suffering from this life threatening disorder and should seek prompt medical attention from your family physician.

- Excessive daytime sleepiness (EDS)
- Morning headaches and/or nausea
- Depression and/or anxiety
- Sexual dysfunction
- Automatic behavior syndrome—behaving automatically in routine tasks and not remembering doing so
- Morning confusion with generalized poor memory
- Sleep walking
- Daytime hallucinations when resisting sleepiness
- Chronic sinus infections
- Exercise intolerance
- Swelling of the feet and ankles
- History of childhood snoring

- A short thick neck with excessive fatty tissue
- Known cardiovascular disease
- Personality changes—aggression, irritability, apathy, impulsiveness, lowered frustration tolerance, jealousy, and suspiciousness

A typical pattern develops in which a person falls asleep and, being unable to breathe during sleep, becomes restless and awakens choking and gasping for air sometimes hundreds of times per night! As the apnea sufferer begins to fall asleep, loud snoring ensues and he begins to experience air hunger: The mouth opens, the chest and abdomen begin heaving, and he frequently thrashes his arms and legs about. Eventually the individual's body becomes exhausted and he or she stops the struggle to breathe and the stage of complete apnea occurs. All body movement ceases and breathing stops until the oxygen level becomes so low the person awakens in order to breathe again. As a result, the apneic individual suffers from severe sleep deprivation and appears chronically lethargic, irritable, and often has difficulty managing daily affairs that others take for granted. The apneic individual suffers from a state of chronic exhaustion and memory impairment. Tragically, family and friends often label the apnea sufferer as lazy or the older adult, senile.

Often the apneic individual is not even aware that he is suffering from this disorder. Although he may be awakening hundreds of times per night to breathe, the level of arousal may not be adequate to produce a fully conscious level of awareness. These partial awakenings result in an interruption of the normal sleep stages necessary for healthy, adaptive functioning. Sleep apnea can have tragic consequences upon a person's self-esteem. Not knowing why he feels the way he does, he often begins to believe other people's simplistic view that he is lazy or in the early stages of senility. What some people may call laziness is in fact a potentially fatal condition that results in severe cardiovascular complications if left untreated.

Two completely different factors may cause sleep apnea, although the presenting symptoms are much the same. First exist the obstructive apneas, which are by far the most common. An obstruction caused by enlarged tonsils or adenoids, a chronic sinus infection, an enlarged tongue, a tumor, or excessive fatty tissue in the neck may be responsible for the symptoms. When the obstructive apnea sufferer is awake, the muscle tone in the breathing passages is usually adequate to bypass the obstructing condition and maintain adequate air exchange. When this person falls asleep, however, and his muscles begin to relax and loosen, the obstructing condition often begins to interfere with normal breathing.

The second form of apnea is called central apnea. This condition occurs when the central nervous system cannot regulate the breathing impulses it sends to the chest and diaphragm muscles. This pattern results in erratic breathing that, as in obstructive apnea, results in a continual interruption of sleep. Finally, more common than pure central apnea, is a garden salad variety of both types of apnea: mixed apnea.

A major indicator of both types of apnea, however, is the loud and thunderous snoring that becomes a source of complaint for all family members. The snoring pattern is characteristic: incredibly loud episodes interrupted by periods of silence. These periods of silence are the apneic nonbreathing cycles which result in severe illness if left untreated. In addition to the characteristic snoring which is always present in sleep apnea, but louder and more robust in obstructive apneas, certain physical traits often present themselves as well. An individual who has a history of snoring, suffers from obesity, has a short, thick neck, and clubbing of fingertips comprise a classic victim of sleep apnea.

Although these may be textbook indicators of this disorder, they are by no means a necessity for diagnosis. Snoring and nonbreathing episodes may be present in normal weight individuals as well, and unfortunately may go undiagnosed because textbook symptomology is not present. If a person complains of constant and vivid dreaming, and feels tired and lethargic throughout the day, suspect sleep apnea. An individual who reports a history of heavy snoring as a child and suffers from high blood pressure as an adult may, too, be suffering from sleep apnea. The point is, various combinations of symptomology may exist, but they can all indicate the same life-threatening condition.

Not only is the apneic individual sleep deprived, but he or she is also oxygen deprived. The shortage of oxygen can become so severe that if left untreated, one can literally die of suffocation. This oxygen deficiency is responsible for the reported morning confusion and memory loss of the victim. In addition, oxygen deprivation produces chronic fatigue, exercise intolerance, anxiety, and morning headaches. With proper treatment, however, apnea victims can once again regain lost energy and their vitality for living.

CARDIOVASCULAR COMPLICATIONS

The irregular breathing patterns that occur during sleep place severe strain on the heart and blood vessels. As a result, apneic individuals have a high occurrence of irregular heartbeat and hypertension, and are at an increased risk for strokes and heart attacks. During periods of nonbreathing, the apneic's blood pressure rises. When breathing resumes, blood pressure returns to normal. In situations where nonbreathing occurs in rapid succession, however, the blood pressure is unable to return to normal. As a result, the individual shows a sustained elevation in nighttime blood pressure. It is common for normal daytime blood pressure to increase to 200/100 or higher during periods of apnea. It becomes obvious, then, that blood pressure this high could damage an individual's cardiovascular system, predisposing him or her to strokes or heart attacks. After suffering years of nighttime hypertension, sleep apnea finally takes its toll and nocturnal hypertension becomes chronic, with sufficient systemic damage to result in full-blown cardiovascular disease. Although the reason remains unclear, this type of intermittent hypertension is more pronounced in obstructive apnea, possibly related to the victims' marked physical struggle to maintain breathing. Those suffering from central apnea appear to struggle less due to the near paralysis of their chest and diaphragm muscles.

In addition to the increase in blood pressure, further damage is done by the fluctuations in heart rate. During nonbreathing periods, it is common for the heart rate to slow to 30 or fewer beats per minute. This is a characteristic pattern in sleep apnea and in severe cases the heart may reverse its action in an attempt to stimulate faster heart action and begin producing extremely weak, rapid, and irregular heartbeats. Unfortunately, this type of cardiac response can be fatal.

Most of an individual's apneic episodes increase during REM sleep when oxygen levels are at their lowest. These nonbreathing episodes, coupled with the lowered oxygen levels that normally occur during REM sleep, comprise the period when most of the cardiovascular damage occurs. Since the longest periods of REM occur during the second half of the night, this is frequently when the greatest damage takes place.

Because apnea sufferers most pronounced difficulties occur during REM periods, the phase of sleep when most dreaming occurs, the apnea victim frequently reports excessive dreaming. Typically, the apneic individual enters REM, begins the normal dreaming process while simultaneously nonbreathing. He awakens to breathe, unlike the normal sleeper and, therefore, remembers the normal and intense dreaming that occurs during this phase of sleep. As a result, the apnea sufferer rarely completes the REM cycle and ends up REM deprived. It is the REM deprivation that accounts for the apneic individual's irritability, impulsivity, hostility, and poor memory.

Sleeping medications also exacerbate symptoms of sleep apnea. Many people suffering from this life-threatening disorder take sleeping aids in effort to gain a restful night's sleep. Unfortunately, many such drugs (including alcohol) depress the central nervous system and interfere with the apneic's ability to awaken to initiate breathing. In addition, these drugs directly influence muscle tone by exaggerating the relaxation effect, weakening the already ineffectual respiratory muscles. These factors can be life threatening, but even if not sufficient to cause death, they certainly produce an increase in oxygen deprivation. This increases the individual's odds for severe cardiovascular complications.

TREATMENT APPROACHES

If you suspect that you may be suffering from sleep apnea or have a history of heavy snoring, it is essential that you seek prompt medical attention. Medical complications may take years to develop but usually become apparent by a person's mid-forties. Don't ignore this problem—you can prevent or significantly reduce the complications that develop with early and appropriate treatment.

Often your bed partner's observations are sufficient for detection of sleep apnea. Effective treatment and management of sleep apnea, however, require the intervention of an accredited sleep disorders program. Typically, when entering such a program, one stays in a sleep lab overnight where clinicians make recordings, called polysomnographs, of heartbeat, brain waves, eye movements, and breathing. You can obtain additional information on reputable sleep centers in or near your area from most major universities, medical schools, or hospitals.

Physicians can correct some obstructive forms of apnea with relatively simple intervention. A weight-reduction program and maintaining a 45 degree elevation of the head and chest during sleep may help mild sleep apnea. For others, however, the condition may require more extensive treatment such as nasal continuous positive airway pressure (CPAP). This treatment model involves wearing a nighttime nasal mask from which compressed air is administered to help maintain an open airway. CPAP is effective in reducing the symptoms of sleep apnea in approximately 75 percent of sufferers.

Chronic sinus infections may also contribute to the development of obstructive apnea. This condition may require treatment by an air, nose, and throat specialist and not over-the-counter decongestants. Finally, in some cases, surgery may be required to remove enlarged adenoids or tonsils, to remove nasal polyps (small tumors with stemlike attachments in the nasal cavity), or for the realignment of the upper and lower jaw.

In the most pronounced cases of sleep apnea, a surgical procedure called an uvulopalatopharyngoplasty (UPPP) may be necessary. An UPPP is a reconstructive procedure in which surgical correction is made to the roof of the mouth, the pharynx, throat area, and uvula. The uvula is the small soft structure hanging from the edge of the soft palate at the top of the esophagus.

The most profound cases of apnea may require a tracheotomy. In this procedure a tube is inserted into a surgical incision in the trachea to bypass tracheal obstructions. Those who require this procedure open the tube at bedtime to enable trouble-free breathing and close it during the day to maintain normal vocal cord action. Although a tracheotomy may sound like an extreme measure, the results produce such a marked improvement in sleep, daytime functioning, and overall health that many individuals feel the treatment is well worth the negative aspects of such a surgical procedure.

Central or mixed apnea, however, appears more responsive to certain medications that have yielded moderately positive results. Although the following medications are not cure-alls, they can provide a degree of relief for some individuals.

The first drug, acetazolamide, better known as progesterone, has known respiratory effects. This particular drug increases a person's respiratory drive, which in turn increases oxygen levels. This medication regimen can, therefore, reduce cardiovascular damage, which is significant for mixed and central apnea sufferers, as their brains' respiratory centers lack the drive to maintain normal breathing during sleep.

The second group of drugs that have shown some measure of success is comprised of tricyclic antidepressants, particularly the antidepressant known as protryptyline. A low-dosage regimen of this particular drug reduces REM sleep. The trycyclic antidepressants, however, do not produce the negative results associated with REM deprivation, namely irritability, impulsivity, and poor memory.

Chapter 11
Sudden Infant Death Syndrome

Sudden Infant Death Syndrome (SIDS), commonly known as crib death, is the infant form of sleep apnea that you read about in chapter 10. It affects full-term and premature infants and is characterized by an abnormality in regulation of the cardiovascular and respiratory centers of the brain. As in adult apnea, a SIDS infant may also have physical obstructions. Abnormalities such as enlarged adenoids, blocked nasal airflow, a relaxed soft palate and tongue, or a soft larynx can contribute to sudden death. Lack of obstructive symptoms of respiratory distress, however, suggest central apnea primarily related to defective control in the brain's respiratory center.

The cause of death, though, as determined during autopsies, is often undetermined and inconclusive. Children who die from SIDS simply fail to rebreathe after an apneic episode, but the actual cause of death remains largely a mystery. Researchers, however, realize that in well over half of these infants subtle changes occurred in their brains and lungs. These subtle but abnormal changes can produce hypoxia, a reduced oxygen intake during inspiration. Also frequently noted is the occurrence of a mild respiratory tract infection at the time of death.

Exactly what causes SIDS remains unknown, but awareness of the knowledge that it does exist may help prevent the tragic loss of an infant's life. In the United States alone, approximately 2 out of every 1,000 live births tragically end in sudden death.

SIDS is the leading cause of death in infants between 1 and 12 months of age, with peak mortality occurring between the ages of two and four months. Sudden death rarely occurs during the first few weeks of life. Typically, babies with mild apnea develop symptoms earlier than infants with more severe types. Symptoms of severe apnea usually begin later, often during the second and third month of life. Unfortunately, if left untreated, 90 percent of SIDS infants die before they reach six months of age.

Many of the SIDS infants grow slowly postnatally even though they were not small for their gestational age. Nor does it appear there is a strong genetic predisposition. There is evidence, however, to suggest the youngest of twins may be at higher risk. It also appears that siblings of a SIDS infant are at greater risk than those in non-SIDS families. In addition, researchers suspect that maternal blood types O and B may increase the risk for SIDS. The reason for this, unfortunately, remains unclear. Ethnicity is also an important factor. In the United States, Orientals are at the lowest risk as opposed to American Indians, Alaskan natives, and Blacks, who have the highest risk factors.

There are certain indicators that predispose an infant to SIDS. These are outlined in the following charts, broken down into pregnancy and infant categories:

Pregnancy History
- Teenage mother
- Drug or alcohol use*
- Cigarette smoking*
- Prior miscarriage
- History of anemia during pregnancy
- Premature delivery*
- History of vaginal infections
- History of protein in urine
- Drop in blood pressure during the third trimester of pregnancy
- Suffered illness (excluding morning sickness)
- Short interpregnancy intervals

(*Major predictors of SIDS)

Infant History
- Required resuscitation at birth
- Received antibiotics postnatally
- Has anemia
- Lives in home where adults smoke
- Develops respiratory infection

- Born premature or has low birth rate
- Is a tremulous infant or has frequent muscle twitching
- Has hypo- or hyper-muscle tone
- Has an abnormal suck and/or difficulty feeding with frequent regurgitation of meals
- Contracts spontaneous fever or hypothermia (often due to extremes in the environment, and/or improper dressing, particularly overwrapping)
- Is non-White—Blacks, American Indians, Alaskan natives
- Is male (two to one occurrence)
- Has an unusual cry (the result of abnormal upper airway muscles, possibly indicating obstructive apnea)
- Is inactive and unresponsive
- Sleeps on a too soft or waterbed mattress (prevents adequate stimulation for respiration)
- Is placed in prone position for sleep.

(Approximately 30 percent of SIDS cases have none of the above findings.)

Most SIDS infants die at night in their sleep, and recent research indicates that deaths may be associated with infants lying in a prone position. Deaths usually occur during winter months with about 50 percent of the babies having had a mild illness the week preceding death. When no immediate illness was present, it is likely that a more severe illness occurred sometime between birth and death. Although not-confirmed studies link abnormalities of the heart to SIDS, studies show that some SIDS-prone infants have elevated sleeping heart rates. As a result, scientists continue to be reluctant to rule out cardiovascular involvement.

CHEMICAL DEPENDENCY

A family member's cigarette smoking may put an infant at risk by causing an alteration in placental and umbilical arteries. This alteration may be the result of the carbon monoxide contained in cigarette smoke. It doesn't take an active imagination to see how smoking could result in impaired cardio/respiratory function in the newborn infant. This is particularly applicable to the Black mother-to-be. For reasons that remain unclear, Black infants seem to be at greater risk when exposed to carbon monoxide than other races.

Also associated with SIDS, but not proven as causal, is maternal narcotic addiction. The infants most susceptible are full-term babies who are small for gestational age. Brain stem regulation in these infants is depressed and remains so well after birth. Since this is the area of the brain that regulates breathing, these babies are prime candidates for apnea and sudden death.

TREATMENT METHODS

Warning: Nonbreathing episodes greater than 10 seconds are approaching the DANGER ZONE.

Remember that infant apnea is life threatening; therefore, you must take any nonbreathing episode as a danger signal. If you suspect that your baby may have had an apneic episode you should take her to an emergency facility immediately. If, on the other hand, she is not breathing and unconscious, call for an ambulance. Until the ambulance arrives, you must employ artificial respiration. To do so, place the infant on her back, turn her head to the side, and check inside her mouth to make sure nothing is obstructing her breathing. Then straighten the infant's head and gently tilt it backward. You then cover her nose and mouth with your mouth and blow 20 short breaths per minute. If you are doing it correctly, you will be able to see your baby's chest gently rise. After each breath lift your mouth away from hers and listen for the sound of returning air. Please note this is just a brief overview of mouth-to-mouth resuscitation technique and is not a substitute for proper training.

If your infant arrives unconscious and unresponsive at the hospital, your family will automatically become part of a SIDS prevention program. This may not be the case, however, if a previously nonbreathing infant arrives at the emergency room alert and responsive. Often these parents believe they may have overreacted. *Don't make this mistake if it happens to you.* Instead, request that hospital personnel refer you to a local SIDS chapter and a pediatrician knowledgeable in infant apnea. A quick reaction is paramount. Although your baby may have spontaneously started rebreathing this time, the next time she may not!

When a physician diagnoses your infant as apneic, he or she will examine your baby to determine whether he has obstructive or central apnea. If central apnea is determined, the physician will likely begin a medication regimen to reduce or eliminate abnormal breathing. When an infant has obstructive apnea, surgical intervention may be necessary.

If an infant has central apnea that does not respond to medication and he is over one month of age, a doctor will recommend electronic monitoring of his heart and respiration rates. However, the monitoring device is not a treatment, nor is it a substitute for well-trained parents. The monitor is merely an alarm to alert parents that their infant is not breathing, or the infant's heart rate is not within the prescribed target zone.

Once parents are part of the SIDS educational and support program they are trained in CPR and monitor management. Through the support of other SIDS families and trained personnel, new parents can develop the ability to stay calm in crises and gain the loving and caring support so needed.

Generally, electronic monitoring can be stopped when an infant reaches eight months and has been apnea free for at least two months. If parents do not seek treatment for their infant, however, there is a 5 percent chance that he will not survive his first nonbreathing episode. If there are additional apneic episodes, the mortality rate increases to roughly 40 percent and climbs even higher if a respiratory infection is present.

Your infant's pediatrician will determine the appropriate treatment regimen based upon his examination results. We do not intend for this information to be a substitute for prompt and thorough diagnosis by a physician. Instead, we hope it serves as an educational tool to increase your level of awareness and alert you to facts that could save the life of your infant.

For further information contact your pediatrician, local SIDS chapter, or the American Red Cross.

Chapter 12
Parenting for Prevention

We decided to end this book with a focus on the beginning. The most important beginning—the beginning of your child's future. We hope this book can help you change habits and patterns that contribute to insomnia, but how much more effective if those same habits and patterns can be prevented in your children. Consistently giving your child the tools he needs to develop strength, confidence, and respect for self and others is the greatest gift he will ever receive. The effects will be far reaching—not only will he sleep easily, but he will embrace life, happy, healthy and equipped to meet life's challenges.

Unfortunately, adults who suffer from insomnia frequently report that their sleeping habits, bedtime rules, and communication patterns with their parents during childhood were inconsistent at best. It is this early inconsistency that lays the groundwork for the development of insomnia during adulthood. There is much that parents can do, however, to prevent their children from developing insomnia, during both childhood and adulthood.

If inconsistency promotes the development of insomnia, consistency is a key to prevent it. As a parent, you can begin to establish healthy sleep habits the first day your infant arrives home from the hospital. Once you have met your baby's needs and put him to bed for a nap or nighttime sleep, resist responding to him if he begins crying. Often this crying is merely a demand for attention. If you pick your baby up every time he or she cries, your infant will quickly learn to associate bed with wakefulness and not with sleep.

Crying is an infant's only means of expressing pain or displeasure and parents should remain alert to respond to their child's needs. A baby, however, can quickly learn to use his crying as a tool for manipulation. A parent that overresponds to a demanding infant's refusal to sleep is paving the path for the development of insomnia later in the child's life.

It is necessary that your baby gets the message within the first few months of life that bed is a place for sleep. It is not a place where he or she can become the victor in a power struggle with Mom or Dad. Not only will this make life easier on you as parents, but your baby will be more content as well.

As a child grows, parents must maintain a consistent bedtime routine. A small child requires 9 or 10 hours of sleep for healthy growth and development and should not, therefore, stay up past 9:00 p.m. Nor should parents allow her to be up roaming about the house by herself before the rest of the family gets up. Even when the young child protests her routine bedtime, you must be firm. A child who learns inconsistent sleep patterns frequently carries these poor sleeping habits into adulthood. Despite a child's complaints, consistency in parenting provides the child with a strong sense of security and well-being.

As a parent, you can maintain bedtime rules and, yet, establish a winding down period for your child that maintains consistency but avoids an unhealthy demand for rigid conformity. Whether you offer 10 to 15 minutes of story time or 15-10-5 minute reminders before bed, a flexible and positive focus on rule enforcement will keep your child happy, relaxed and free of resentment—all prerequisites for a great night's sleep.

DIET

Because a child's delicate system arouses easily, parents must avoid all stimulating food or drink at least four hours before bedtime. Parents should refrain from giving their children any foods containing caffeine or sugar (such as chocolate, soda, tea, or ice cream) after the evening meal. Vitamin supplements can also prove stimulating for some children. Do not give them any vitamins at bedtime, but instead with the child's morning meal.

STRESS RESPONSE

Although poor sleep habits set the stage for sleeplessness, stress is frequently the trigger that sets insomnia in motion. As a parent, you must recognize and respect, therefore, that a child's feelings are as intense as yours. Stress affects all children profoundly. Parents console their children when they are exposed to divorce, family arguments, or the loss of a beloved pet, for example, but usually avoid actively discussing the problem itself. Unfortunately, in an attempt to protect their children, parents often end up adding to their confusion. You need to address the stressful situation in a supportive way that is age-appropriate to help your child process the information and reduce his stress level.

A child develops his coping style by observing the significant people in his life. Although observation can be an excellent learning tool for children, observation alone can often produce distorted learning experiences for them, particularly when they do not understand the nature of what they are observing. Although providing a child with all the details of a situation may not be appropriate, you should offer an edited version. This dispels the confusion that a child feels because he is uninformed. By discussing the feelings that accompany stress, a child can gain an understanding of the emotions he has in association with the situation.

When we try to avoid communicating with our children about family stressors, they pick up on the emotional climate. Coupled with the confusion this produces, these children cannot learn to express emotion appropriately because there is always an element of confusion associated with their feelings. If we do not give them the opportunity to discuss a situation, they will not learn how to verbalize or work through their feelings. As a result, they grow into adults who have difficulty expressing or understanding their emotions.

A child, therefore, needs to experience the good and bad that life has to offer. Guided by caring parents, she can learn that true resolution of a crisis involves dealing with it—and not denying or avoiding the painful emotions that accompany it. Children who are overly protected become fearful adults who lack the ability to understand or express their emotion. Expression continues, nevertheless, and often surfaces in the guise of ulcers, insomnia, or hypertension.

When we discourage our children from expressing emotion, they grow into adults who are not in touch with their feelings, or, worse yet, deny having any at all. And a well-meaning parent can innocently accomplish this by urging his child to be strong when he needs to cry, or trying to resolve his personal crisis by telling him, "Everything will be alright, don't worry." Children need to communicate if they are to adjust well to life. If they do not communicate verbally, they will communicate through confusing avenues such as bed-wetting, sleepwalking, nightmares, or childhood onset insomnia.

As a parent, you can help prevent these problems from developing by encouraging your child to clarify her emotions. A parent can help a young child sort through and learn to recognize and understand emotions she may not yet be able to label. Learning to read or learning one's multiplication tables requires practice and guidance from an experienced teacher; so, too, does learning to understand one's emotions. As an adult, you can assume the role of teacher and counselor. You can provide your child with the necessary instruction to enable her to gain an understanding of herself. A child who learns to understand her emotions will likewise learn to accept and trust her emotional interpretation of events as an adult.

Although assurance and consolation are necessary parts of parenting, you need to take this one step further and actively communicate with your child. A child can often be a master of emotional disguise, so don't wait for him to approach you, because he may not. Observe your child for signs of stress and realize that if you as a parent are experiencing tension, it is quite likely that your daughter or son is also. Talk to your child and ask what he feels like inside. Then discuss what feelings are appropriate for a given situation and how emotions such as happiness and anger differ from one another. Teach him that anger, pain, and sorrow are not diseases, but are part of what defines him; that they are not constant and fixed, but can instead serve as motivation to help him successfully resolve conflict in his life through change or acceptance. You can help him realize that his feelings are nothing he should fear. Instead, they are a valuable tool in helping him understand himself, interpret situations, and appropriately meet his needs.

In addition to establishing firm bedtime rules, you must actively communicate with your child about the stress in his life and the family's life. Help him clarify, express, and accept his emotions because, by doing so, he will be less likely to develop emotional and physical illnesses not only during childhood, but throughout his entire lifetime.

Appendix
Thought Journal

Automatic thoughts: _____

_____

_____

_____

Distorted thoughts: _____

_____

_____

_____

Associated feelings: _____

_____

_____

Rational thoughts: _____

_____

_____

Thought errors: _____

_____

_____

_____

Origin of thought: _____

_____

_____

_____

Index